Infectious Diseases and Microbiology

snova
New York

Infectious Diseases and Microbiology

Diseases Transmitted by Ticks
Hacer İşler (Editor)
Metin Özdemir, MD (Editor)
2021. ISBN: 978-1-68507-359-6 (Hardcover)
2021. ISBN: 978-1-68507-383-1 (eBook)

Impacts and Implications of COVID-19: An Analytical and Empirical Study
Anand Sharma (Editor)
Prateek Agrawal (Editor)
Vishu Madaan (Editor)
Anuj Agarwal (Editor)
2021. ISBN: 978-1-53619-670-2 (Hardcover)
2021. ISBN: 978-1-68507-081-6 (eBook)

Understanding the Spread of Infectious Diseases
Andrew J. Hinerman (Editor)
2020. ISBN: 978-1-53618-892-9 (Hardcover)
2020. ISBN: 978-1-53618-917-9 (eBook)

COVID-19 Pandemic: Questions, Answers and Hypotheses
A.K. Haghi (Editor)
2020. ISBN: 978-1-53618-565-2 (Softcover)
2020. ISBN: 978-1-53618-593-5 (eBook)

COVID 19
Sujith Ovallath, MBBS, MD, DNB, DM (Author)
2020. ISBN: 978-1-53618-691-8 (Softcover)
2020. ISBN: 978-1-53618-729-8 (eBook)

More information about this series can be found at
https://novapublishers.com/product-category/series/infectious-diseases-and-microbiology-new-in-2020/

Eric Neudorf
Editor

COVID-19 Contracting

Opportunities, Actions and Reimbursements

New York

Library of Congress Cataloging-in-Publication Data

ISBN: 978-1-68507-710-5

Published by Nova Science Publishers, Inc. † New York

Contents

Preface vii

Chapter 1 **COVID-19 Contracting: Opportunities to Improve Practices to Assess Prospective Vendors and Capture Lessons Learned** 1
United States Government Accountability Office

Chapter 2 **COVID-19 Contracting: Actions Needed to Enhance Transparency and Oversight of Selected Awards** 73
United States Government Accountability Office

Chapter 3 **COVID-19 Contracting: Contractor Paid Leave Reimbursements Could Provide Lessons Learned for Future Emergency Responses** 147
United States Government Accountability Office

Chapter 4 **COVID-19 Contracting: Indian Health Service Used Flexibilities to Meet Increased Medical Supply Needs** 175
United States Government Accountability Office

Index 197

Preface

In March 2020, Congress passed the CARES Act as part of the federal response to COVID-19. The act had certain provisions for federal contracting, including providing additional flexibilities. Contracting plays a critical role in the pandemic response as agencies obligate billions of dollars for goods and services.

The act also included a provision to review federal contracting in response to COVID-19. This book examines, among other objectives, COVID-19 contract obligations and characteristics of vendors, contracting challenges, including with agency assessments of vendors, and whether lessons learned efforts reflect those challenges.

Chapter 1 - In response to COVID-19, agencies awarded contracts for goods and services to vendors from a range of industries and with varying levels of federal contracting experience, but some vendors have been unable to deliver under those contracts.

The CARES Act included a provision for GAO to review COVID-19-related federal contracting under the act. This report addresses (1) COVID-19 contract obligations and characteristics of vendors, (2) contracting challenges, including with agency assessments of vendors, and (3) whether lessons learned efforts reflect those challenges.

GAO analyzed federal procurement data on agencies' reported COVID-19 contract obligations through May 31, 2021. GAO examined a nongeneralizable sample of 28 contracts with high dollar values or other characteristics from four agencies—DOD, HHS, USDA, and DHS. GAO interviewed officials, including Office of Management and Budget (OMB) officials about their emergency acquisition guidance.

Chapter 2 - In March 2020, Congress passed the CARES Act as part of the federal response to COVID-19. The act had certain provisions for federal contracting, including providing additional flexibilities. Contracting plays a critical role in the pandemic response as agencies obligate billions of dollars for goods and services.

The act also included a provision for GAO to review federal contracting in response to COVID-19. This report examines, among other objectives, the extent to which the Departments of Defense, Health and Human Services, and Homeland Security—the only agencies that reported using other transaction agreements in response to COVID-19 in the federal procurement database—used such agreements, including awards to consortia, and oversight of such use.

GAO analyzed federal procurement data as of March 2021; reviewed a nongeneralizable sample of 15 agreements selected based on high dollar amounts, agency, a mix of products and services, among other criteria; reviewed agency policies; and interviewed agency officials.

Chapter 3 - In March 2020, Congress passed the CARES Act, which provides over $2 trillion in emergency assistance for those affected by COVID-19.

Section 3610 of the CARES Act enables agencies, at their discretion, to reimburse contractors for paid leave provided to their employees and subcontractors who are unable to access work sites due to facility closures or other restrictions, and whose duties cannot be performed remotely during the pandemic. The CARES Act also includes a provision for GAO to review federal contracting pursuant to authorities provided in the Act.

In September 2020, GAO found that agencies had not made much use of section 3610 authority as of July 2020, and expectations of future use varied.

This report (1) examines how selected federal agencies have used section 3610 authority and (2) presents selected contractors' perspectives on COVID-19 paid leave reimbursement. GAO reviewed guidance and data and interviewed cognizant officials from four agencies with contract obligations greater than $10 billion in fiscal year 2019. GAO also selected a non-generalizable sample of 15 contractors that received or requested section 3610 reimbursements from one or more of the selected agencies and conducted semi-structured interviews of contractor representatives.

Chapter 4 - The Indian Health Service (IHS) serves over 2 million American Indians and Alaska Natives. These groups have been disproportionately vulnerable to negative outcomes from COVID-19. During emergencies, federal contracting staff face pressure to work quickly to meet increased needs. We examined some of IHS's COVID- related contracts to see how the agency's efforts fared.

Chapter 1

COVID-19 Contracting: Opportunities to Improve Practices to Assess Prospective Vendors and Capture Lessons Learned*

United States Government Accountability Office

Abbreviations

AMS	Agricultural Marketing Service
ASPR	Office of the Assistant Secretary for Preparedness and Response
BARDA	Biomedical Advanced Research and Development Authority
COVID-19	Coronavirus Disease 2019
CPARS	Contractor Performance Assessment Reporting System
DHS	Department of Homeland Security
DLA	Defense Logistics Agency
DOD	Department of Defense
E2A2	Exercise, Evaluation and After Actions Division
FAPIIS	Federal Awardee Performance and Integrity Information System
FAR	Federal Acquisition Regulation
FEMA	Federal Emergency Management Agency
FPDS	Federal Procurement Data System
HHS	Department of Health and Human Services

* This is an edited, reformatted and augmented version of the United States Government Accountability Office Report to Congressional Addressees, Publication No. GAO-21-528, dated July 2021.

In: COVID-19 Contracting
Editor: Eric Neudorf
ISBN: 978-1-68507-710-5

OFPP	Office of Federal Procurement Policy
OMB	Office of Management and Budget
SAM	System for Award Management
USACE	U.S. Army Corps of Engineers
USDA	U.S. Department of Agriculture

Why GAO Did This Study

In response to COVID-19, agencies awarded contracts for goods and services to vendors from a range of industries and with varying levels of federal contracting experience, but some vendors have been unable to deliver under those contracts.

The CARES Act included a provision for GAO to review COVID-19-related federal contracting under the act. This report addresses (1) COVID-19 contract obligations and characteristics of vendors, (2) contracting challenges, including with agency assessments of vendors, and (3) whether lessons learned efforts reflect those challenges.

GAO analyzed federal procurement data on agencies' reported COVID-19 contract obligations through May 31, 2021. GAO examined a nongeneralizable sample of 28 contracts with high dollar values or other characteristics from four agencies—DOD, HHS, USDA, and DHS. GAO interviewed officials, including Office of Management and Budget (OMB) officials about their emergency acquisition guidance.

What GAO Recommends

GAO is making 10 recommendations, including that agencies establish processes to better collect and communicate contracting lessons learned during emergencies such as COVID-19. Agencies agreed with nine recommendations. OMB did not agree to establish time frames for updating its guidance. GAO continues to believe OMB should do so, as discussed in this report.

What GAO Found

As of May 31, 2021, agencies obligated $61.4 billion for contracts in response to the COVID-19 pandemic. Agencies cancelled $4 billion in obligations, in some cases due to contract terminations. The proportion of obligations to vendors with prior federal experience government-wide was 88 percent but varied by agency (see figure). In calendar year 2020, agencies awarded about 5 times as many contracts to vendors without prior federal contracting experience for COVID-19, as compared to contracts awarded overall in preceding calendar years.

COVID-19-Related Contract Obligations to Vendors with or without Prior Federal Contracting Experience for the Five Agencies with the Most Obligations, as of May 31, 2021

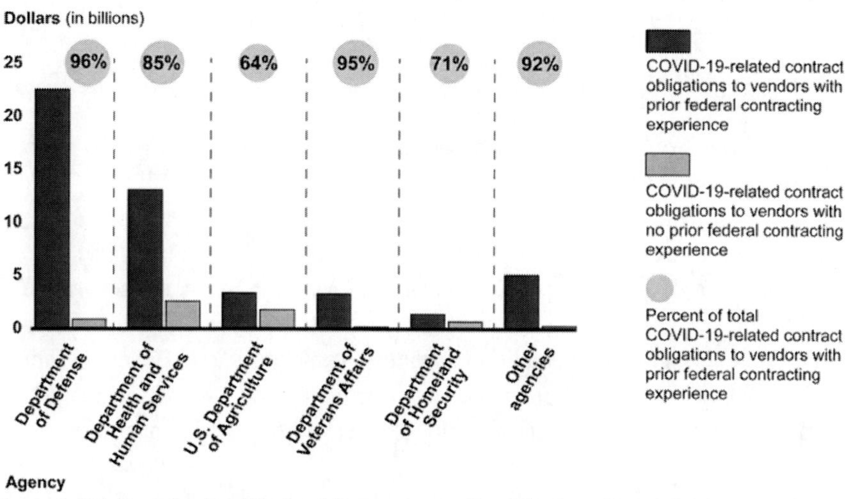

Source: GAO analysis of Federal Procurement Data System data. | GAO-21-528.

For the selected contracts GAO reviewed across four agencies—the Departments of Defense (DOD), Health and Human Services (HHS), Agriculture (USDA), and Homeland Security (DHS)—contracting officials identified a number of challenges, including:

- working with vendors new to federal contracting or vendors supplying products they had not previously provided;
- operating under limited time frames to make awards; and

- contracting for supplies and services the agency does not typically buy.

The four agencies are collecting and sharing lessons learned related to their COVID-19 response. However, HHS and DHS have not included contracting lessons learned, even though they identified contracting challenges. Collecting contracting lessons learned could inform future emergency response efforts.

Furthermore, although interagency coordination was critical to the response, contracting lessons learned are at risk of not being reflected in formal interagency lessons learned efforts. Without a process to do so, federal agencies risk missing an opportunity to memorialize contracting and coordination practices that were successful, as well as those that were not, for future emergencies.

July 29, 2021
Congressional Addressees

Since the declaration of Coronavirus Disease 2019 (COVID-19) as a national emergency on March 13, 2020, the United States has reported more than 30 million confirmed cases, and there have been significant effects from the pandemic on public health and the economy. To help mitigate these effects, agencies awarded contracts to thousands of vendors from a wide range of industries and with varying levels of federal contracting experience for critical goods and services, such as N95 respirators, ventilators, and the development and production of vaccines. However, during the course of the pandemic, some vendors have been unable to deliver those goods and services as promised.

Our prior work found that contracts play a key role in federal emergency response efforts, and that contracting during an emergency can present a unique set of challenges as officials endeavor to provide critical goods and services as expeditiously and efficiently as possible.[1] For example, our work following the 2017 and 2018 hurricanes and wildfires identified challenges

---

[1] GAO, Disaster Contracting: FEMA Continues to Face Challenges with Its Use of Contracts to Support Response and Recovery, GAO-19-518T (Washington, D.C.: May 9, 2019); 2017 Disaster Contracting: Actions Needed to Improve the Use of Post-Disaster Contracts to Support Response and Recovery, GAO-19-281 (Washington, D.C.: Apr. 24, 2019); and 2017 Disaster Contracting: Action Needed to Better Ensure More Effective Use and Management of Advance Contracts, GAO-19-93 (Washington, D.C: Dec. 6, 2018).

managing, planning, and executing contracts and monitoring purchase card use.[2] These challenges were due, in part, to shortcomings in agency contracting guidance and in efforts to assess fraud risks in a disaster response environment. We have also reported on challenges agencies face identifying and sharing interagency contracting lessons learned following an emergency to improve future response efforts.[3]

The CARES Act included a provision for GAO to provide a comprehensive audit and review of federal contracting pursuant to authorities provided in the act.[4] This report is one in a series of reports examining federal agencies' contracting in response to COVID-19.[5] This report examines (1) contract obligations and characteristics of vendors; (2) the information selected agencies used to assess prospective vendors and the extent to which the agencies communicated available information to contracting officers; and (3) the extent to which selected agencies experienced challenges and established processes to collect and share contracting lessons learned.

To identify contract obligations and characteristics of vendors involved in the response to the COVID-19 pandemic, we analyzed data available in the Federal Procurement Data System (FPDS) as of May 31, 2021.

Though agencies may obligate dollars through various other vehicles such as grants or cooperative agreements, this report is focused specifically on contract obligations.[6] We primarily identified these contract actions and

---

[2] GAO, Disaster Response: Agencies Should Assess Contracting Workforce Needs and Purchase Card Fraud Risk, GAO-21-42 (Washington, D.C.: Nov. 24, 2020); GAO-19-281; and GAO-19-93.

[3] GAO-19-281.

[4] Pub. L. No. 116-136, div. B, tit. IX, § 19010, 134 Stat. 281, 579 (2020). We regularly issue government-wide reports on the federal response to COVID-19. For the latest report, see GAO, COVID-19: Continued Attention Needed to Enhance Federal Preparedness, Response, Service Delivery, and Program Integrity, GAO-21-551 (Washington, D.C.: July 19, 2021). Our next government-wide report will be issued in October 2021 and will be available on GAO's website at https://www.gao.gov/coronavirus.

[5] 5GAO, COVID-19 Contracting: Contractor Paid Leave Reimbursements Could Provide Lessons Learned for Future Emergency Response, GAO-21-475, (Washington, D.C.: July 28, 2021); COVID-19 Contracting: Actions Needed to Enhance Transparency and Oversight of Selected Awards, GAO-21-501 (Washington, D.C.: July 26, 2021); Defense Production Act: Opportunities Exist to Increase Transparency and Identify Future Actions to Mitigate Medical Supply Chain Issues, GAO-21-108 (Washington, D.C.: Nov. 19, 2020); COVID-19 Contracting: Observations on Contractor Paid Leave Reimbursement Guidance and Use, GAO-20-662 (Washington, D.C.: Sept. 3, 2020); and COVID-19 Contracting: Observations on Federal Contracting in Response to the Pandemic, GAO-20-632 (Washington, D.C.: July 29, 2020).

[6] For the purposes of this report, "contract obligations" means obligations on contracts that are subject to the Federal Acquisition Regulation, and does not include, for example, grants,

associated obligations related to the COVID-19 response by using the National Interest Action code.[7] We took additional steps to ensure contract actions and obligations included in our analysis were related to COVID-19. For a detailed description of these actions, see appendix I. We assessed the reliability of FPDS data by reviewing existing information about the system and the data it collects— specifically, the data dictionary and validation rules—and performing electronic testing. We determined the FPDS data were sufficiently reliable for the purposes of describing agencies' reported contract obligations to vendors in response to COVID-19.

We analyzed the FPDS data to identify the agencies with the highest COVID-19 contract obligations, the types of goods and services procured, and vendor characteristics, such as whether a vendor had prior federal contracting experience and whether the vendor was a small or large business. We augmented data from FPDS with data from the System for Award Management (SAM) and the Federal Awardee Performance and Integrity Information System (FAPIIS) to identify additional information about vendors receiving COVID-19 contracts. This information included whether or not vendors were registered in SAM and whether or not there was a record in FAPIIS identifying prior performance or integrity concerns.

To determine what information selected agencies used to assess prospective vendors that were awarded contracts in response to COVID- 19, we selected four of the top five departments with the highest COVID- 19 contract obligations as of August 31, 2020—the Departments of Defense (DOD), Health and Human Services (HHS), Agriculture (USDA), and Homeland Security (DHS).[8] Within these departments, we selected the agencies that collectively accounted for at least two-thirds of each department's COVID-19 contract obligations:

---

cooperative agreements, loans, other transactions for research, real property leases, or requisitions from federal stock.

[7] National Interest Action codes were established in 2005 after Hurricane Katrina with the purpose of tracking federal procurements for specific disasters, emergencies, or contingency events. A National Interest Action code was established on March 13, 2020, for the COVID-19 pandemic, and contract actions and their associated obligations are coded as related to the COVID-19 response in a field in FPDS.

[8] We selected August 31, 2020 as it was the time we were beginning and scoping our review. The other agency with the highest contract obligations was the Department of Veterans Affairs, which we did not include due to other ongoing work on the department's contracting response to COVID-19. See GAO, VA COVID-19 Procurements: Pandemic Underscores Urgent Need to Modernize Supply Chain, GAO-21-280 (Washington, D.C.: June 15, 2021).

- DOD's Defense Logistics Agency (DLA) and Department of the Army;
- HHS's Office of the Assistant Secretary for Preparedness and Response (ASPR);
- USDA's Agricultural Marketing Service (AMS); and
- DHS's Federal Emergency Management Agency (FEMA).

We collected and reviewed contract files for a nongeneralizable sample of 28 contracts and task or delivery orders (hereafter referred to as contracts, unless otherwise specified), seven from each department awarded between January 2020 and August 31, 2020.[9] We selected the contracts based on a variety of factors, including dollar amount and whether the contract was awarded to a vendor with prior federal contracting experience.[10] For our selected contracts, we gathered and reviewed contract documentation related to agency assessments of prospective vendors' responsibility and capability, such as vendor proposals, responsibility determinations (where available), and source selection evaluation reports. We also conducted semi-structured interviews with contracting officials responsible for the 28 selected contracts to discuss the resources they used to assess prospective vendors.

To assess the extent to which selected agencies communicated available information to contracting officers to assess prospective vendors, we reviewed agency, department, and government-wide guidance and regulations related to assessing prospective vendors and emergency acquisitions. This included the Federal Acquisition Regulation (FAR), department and agency supplements to the FAR, agency guidance and job aids, and the Office of Federal Procurement Policy's (OFPP) Emergency Acquisitions Guide. We also reviewed federal internal control standards on risk assessment, information, and communication.[11] We interviewed acquisition policy and contracting officials responsible for our selected contracts to determine the contracting officers' awareness of information and resources available to assess

---

[9] For DOD, we selected three contracts from DLA and four from the Department of the Army. Within the Department of the Army, we selected one contract from Army Contracting Command and three contracts from the U.S. Army Corps of Engineers.

[10] We initially selected eight contracts and task orders per department for a total of 32 contracts. However, we removed three contracts because they were potentially the subject of an ongoing Office of Inspector General or other federal investigation. We also removed one contract that was reported as awarded in FPDS, but that agency officials told us had, in fact, never been awarded.

[11] GAO, Standards for Internal Control in the Federal Government, GAO-14-704G (Washington, D.C.: September 2014).

prospective vendors during an emergency. We also interviewed OFPP staff to identify efforts, if any, underway to update or revise the Emergency Acquisitions Guide.

To determine the extent to which selected agencies experienced challenges when contracting in response to COVID-19 and established processes to collect and share contracting lessons learned, we interviewed DOD, HHS, USDA, and DHS contracting officials for our 28 selected contracts. We reviewed available COVID-19 after-action reports at DOD, USDA, and DHS to identify agencies' lessons learned and proposed actions to address these lessons.[12] We also interviewed contracting officials at each agency or department and officials responsible for gathering and reporting on lessons learned to assess their efforts to collect and share lessons against leading practices GAO and others have previously identified.[13] Appendix I provides more information about our scope and methodology.

We conducted this performance audit from August 2020 to July 2021 in accordance with generally accepted government auditing standards.

Those standards require that we plan and perform the audit to obtain sufficient, appropriate evidence to provide a reasonable basis for our findings and conclusions based on our audit objectives. We believe that the evidence obtained provides a reasonable basis for our findings and conclusions based on our audit objectives.

---

[12] HHS had not completed an after-action report at the time of our review.

[13] GAO, Army Modernization: Army Should Improve Use of Alternative Agreements and Approaches by Enhancing Oversight and Communication of Lessons Learned, GAO-21-8 (Washington, D.C.: Oct. 1, 2020); DOD Utilities Privatization: Improved Data Collection and Lessons Learned Archive Could Help Reduce Time to Award Contracts, GAO-20-104 (Washington, D.C.: Apr. 2, 2020); Project Management: DOE and NNSA Should Improve Their Lessons-Learned Process for Capital Asset Projects, GAO-19-25 (Washington, D.C.: Dec. 21, 2018); and Federal Real Property Security: Interagency Security Committee Should Implement a Lessons-Learned Process, GAO-12-901 (Washington, D.C.: Sept. 10, 2012). GAO-19-25 identified some lessons learned practices from reports by both the Project Management Institute and Department of the Army, Combined Arms Center, Center for Army Lessons Learned. Project Management Institute, Inc., A Guide to the Project Management Body of Knowledge (PMBOK® Guide), Sixth Edition, 2017; Project Management Institute, Inc., Implementing Organizational Project Management: A Practice Guide, First Edition, 2014; and Center for Army Lessons Learned, Establishing a Lessons Learned Program: Observations, Insights, and Lessons (Fort Leavenworth, KS: June 2011). PMBOK is a trademark of Project Management Institute, Inc.

Background

Agencies have contracted to obtain the goods and services needed to respond to COVID-19 within the context of their specific roles and responsibilities. According to DHS's National Response Framework—a guide to how the federal government, states and localities, and other public and private sector institutions should respond to disasters and emergencies—the Secretary of Homeland Security is responsible for ensuring that federal preparedness actions during a national emergency are coordinated to prevent gaps in the federal government's response.[14] The framework designates FEMA to lead the coordination of disaster response efforts across federal agencies. FEMA coordinates disaster response efforts through mission assignments—work orders that FEMA issues to direct other federal agencies to use the authorities and the resources granted to it under federal law. Mission assignments are authorized by the Robert T. Stafford Disaster Relief and Emergency Assistance Act and can consist of federal operations support or direct federal assistance, which includes federal contracts.[15] During the response to COVID-19, HHS was designated as the lead federal agency to address the public health and medical portion of the response, and FEMA was designated to co-lead the overall federal response.

Federal agencies are designated as coordinating agencies across 15 Emergency Support Functions—specific functional areas for the most frequently needed capabilities during an emergency. The National Response Framework states that when an Emergency Support Function is activated in response to an incident, the primary agency and other support agencies for that emergency support function are responsible for delivering core capabilities that can include contracting. For example:

- The U.S. Army Corps of Engineers (USACE) within DOD is responsible for the provision of assets and services related to public works and engineering. To fulfill this role during the response to COVID-19, the agency awarded contracts for the construction of alternate care facilities to treat COVID-19 patients.[16] In addition, DLA has a standing arrangement with FEMA to acquire goods and

---

[14] Department of Homeland Security, *National Response Framework* (October 2019).

[15] See 42 U.S.C. § 5192(a)(1).

[16] An alternate care facility is a facility that is temporarily converted for health care use during a public health emergency to reduce the burden on hospitals and established medical facilities.

services, and received mission assignments to contract for personal protective equipment like gloves, surgical masks, and gowns in support of the pandemic response.

- HHS is the coordinating agency responsible for public health and medical services, which can include the assessment of public health and medical needs, provision of medical equipment and supplies, and public health communication, among other responsibilities. Within HHS, ASPR leads the nation's medical and public health preparedness for, response to, and recovery from disasters and public health emergencies. ASPR awarded contracts for a variety of COVID-19 medical response needs, including vaccine manufacturing capacity and medical equipment and supplies such as ventilators, N95 respirators, and gloves to replenish the Strategic National Stockpile. Rebuilding the stockpile, which is designed to supplement state and local supplies during public health emergencies, falls under ASPR's responsibilities.
- USDA is the coordinating agency for agriculture and natural resources, which includes functions to protect the nation's food supply and provide nutrition assistance through programs like the Farmers to Families Food Box Program. AMS implemented the Farmers to Families Food Box program in May 2020 to assist commodity suppliers affected by the pandemic and provide food assistance to the public. Through the program, AMS contracted with hundreds of distributors to purchase billions of dollars in fresh fruits, vegetables, dairy, and meat products. These products were then packaged into family-sized food boxes for delivery to food banks, community and faith based organizations, and other non-profit entities around the country.

Given the unprecedented nature of the response to COVID-19, some federal agencies relied on interagency agreements to obtain needed supplies or services from another agency. For example, in April 2020, ASPR established memorandums of understanding with DOD and FEMA for those agencies to provide contracting services and support for the acquisition of medical supplies and services. These supplies and services included personal protective equipment, testing supplies, and construction and renovation of facilities for the production of vaccines and therapeutics. Under the memorandums of understanding, ASPR provided the acquisition requirements to DOD or FEMA, which then contracted for the supply or service, and were subsequently reimbursed by HHS pursuant to the Economy Act.[17]

FAR Requirements Related to Assessing Prospective Vendors

The FAR requires that agencies take certain steps before awarding contracts to prospective vendors:

Contractor responsibility determinations. The FAR requires that no purchase or award be made from a prospective vendor unless the contracting officer has made an affirmative determination of responsibility.[18] To be determined responsible, a prospective contractor must:

- have adequate financial resources to perform the contract, or the ability to obtain them;
- be able to comply with the required or proposed delivery or performance schedule;
- have a satisfactory performance record;
- have a satisfactory record of integrity and business ethics;
- have the necessary organization, experience, accounting and operational controls, and technical skills, or the ability to obtain them;
- have the necessary production, construction, and technical equipment and facilities, or the ability to obtain them; and
- be otherwise qualified and eligible to receive an award under applicable laws and regulations.[19]

In general, the determination of a prospective contractor's responsibility is within the broad discretion of the contracting officer, and contracting officers may collect or review a variety of information to assess a particular element of contractor responsibility. Financial capability, for instance, may be assessed by reviewing documentation from a vendor's lender about their line of credit or by reviewing the vendor's financial statements. Contracting officers have less flexibility in some of the other resources used to assess prospective vendors. For example, the FAR requires contracting officers to

[17] Economy Act, 31 U.S.C. §§ 1535-1536. The Economy Act authorizes agencies to enter into agreements for the interagency provision of goods and services.

[18] FAR § 9.103(b).

[19] FAR § 9.104-1.

review the performance and integrity information available in certain government-wide databases when determining contractor responsibility. Specifically:

- *Federal Awardee Performance and Integrity Information System (FAPIIS):* FAPIIS is designed to assist contracting officers with making a responsibility determination by providing integrity and performance information on federal contractors. Specifically, FAPIIS provides a prospective contractor "Report Card" that includes information pertaining to the contractor's past performance on government contracts (if applicable). This information includes nonresponsibility determinations, exclusions, and, if a contract wasterminated, whether the termination was considered to be at the fault of the contractor.[20] Before awarding any contract over the simplified acquisition threshold, a contracting officer must review prospective contractor's performance and integrity information in FAPIIS and document in the contract file how the information in FAPIIS was used to determine responsibility.[21]
- *System for Award Management (SAM):* SAM is managed by the General Services Administration and is the primary government repository for prospective federal awardee information. Subject to certain exceptions, a vendor must be registered in SAM to comply with mandatory reporting requirements, which can include providing ownership, business size, and tax liability information. The exceptions include contracts awarded without full and open competition due to unusual and compelling urgency and contracts

[20] Contractors may be determined nonresponsible if they do not have a satisfactory record of performance, integrity, or business ethics. For example, failing to make a sufficient effort to perform acceptably on a prior contract is strong evidence of nonresponsibility.
According to SAM, exclusions identify those parties excluded from receiving federal contracts, certain subcontracts, and from certain types of federal financial and non-financial assistance and benefits, and they are also commonly known as "suspensions" and "debarments."

[21] FAR § 9.104-6. Agencies generally must use simplified acquisition procedures for purchases of goods or services at or below the simplified acquisition threshold. The simplified acquisition threshold generally is $250,000, but it increases to $800,000 for acquisitions in the U.S. determined by the head of the agency to support a response to an emergency or major disaster declared under the Robert T. Stafford Disaster Relief and Emergency Assistance Act. FAR § 2.101.

awarded in emergency operations, such as responses to national emergencies like COVID- 19.[22]

- *Contractor Performance Assessment Reporting System (CPARS):* CPARS is an evaluation reporting tool for all past performance reports on government contracts and orders. Past performance reports in CPARS reflect ratings and supporting narratives for various factors, including quality of goods and services, management and business relations, and adherence to schedules. Agencies are generally required to prepare performance evaluations on contracts and orders at least annually, and when the work under a contract is completed.[23]

Vendors that are new to federal contracting may not have information reported in the government's databases. The FAR instructs agencies to conduct, to the maximum extent practicable, market research on an ongoing basis to effectively identify the capabilities of small businesses and new entrants into federal contracting that are available to meet agency requirements for disaster or emergency relief activities, among other things.[24]

While documents and reports supporting a determination of responsibility, such as the use of FAPIIS, must be included in the contract file, the contracting officer's signature on a contract constitutes the determination that a prospective vendor is responsible with respect to the contract.

Source selection. The FAR describes several contracting methods that can vary based on the circumstances of the procurement. For example, a request for proposals is used in negotiated procurements to communicate the government's requirements to prospective vendors and to solicit proposals.[25] Following the receipt of proposals in competitive negotiated procurements, agencies are responsible for evaluating the proposals based solely on the factors and significant subfactors identified in the solicitation. While the selection of these factors and their relative importance are at the discretion of

[22] FAR § 4.1102(a)(3), (5). For contracts awarded in emergency operations, the FAR instructs contracting officers to modify, if practical, the contract to require SAM registration, FAR § 4.1102(b).

[23] FAR § 42.1502(a).

[24] FAR § 10.001(a)(2)(vi).

[25] FAR § 15.203(a). At a minimum, requests for proposals for competitive negotiated procurements must describe the government's requirement, the anticipated terms and conditions that will apply to the contract, the information required to be in the prospective vendor's proposal, and the factors and significant subfactors that will be used to evaluate the proposal and their relative importance.

agency acquisition officials, price or cost, the quality of the good or service, and past performance are generally required to be evaluated in competitive negotiated procurements.[26] For example, regarding proposal evaluation for negotiated procurements, the FAR states that past performance is one indicator of a prospective vendor's ability to successfully perform the contract, and that prospective vendors without a record of relevant past performance cannot be evaluated favorably or unfavorably on that basis.[27]

Agency Regulations and Guidance

Agencies may issue agency-specific acquisition regulations and internal guidance that implements or supplements the FAR.[28] For example, DHS relies on the Homeland Security Acquisition Regulation and Homeland Security Acquisition Manual—issued by DHS's Chief Procurement Officer—to implement and supplement the FAR. Together, these documents provide more specific department-wide policies and procedures for implementing acquisition requirements laid out by the FAR, such as competition, acquisition planning, and market research.

Similarly, within DOD, the Defense Federal Acquisition Regulation Supplement implements and supplements the FAR, and the companion Procedures, Guidance, and Information contains mandatory and non-mandatory internal procedures and guidance. In addition to these resources, DLA and the Department of the Army rely on the Defense Logistics Acquisition Directive and Army Federal Acquisition Regulation Supplement, respectively, to further implement and supplement federal and DOD-wide acquisition regulations. Subject to certain authorities, agencies may issue internal guidance at any organizational level to designate and delegate authorities, assign responsibilities, and identify internal reporting requirements.[29] For example, FEMA's contracting activity issued a Disaster Contracting Desk Guide that it uses internally to supplement the emergency acquisition process and ensure its contracting staff are equipped with the necessary information to conduct its mission.

---

[26] FAR § 15.304(c).

[27] FAR § 15.305(a)(2).

[28] Whether agencies communicate information in internal guidance will depend on the agencies' determination that legal requirements do not necessitate more formal regulations.

[29] See FAR § 1.301(a)(2).

Government-wide, OFPP provides overall direction for procurement policies, regulations, and procedures, and promotes economy, efficiency, and effectiveness in acquisition processes. For example, OFPP issued an Emergency Acquisitions Guide to supplement agency specific guidance and to be used in conjunction with the FAR and the National Response Framework.[30] The guide is intended to assist the federal contracting community with planning and executing procurement activities during contingency operations, major disaster declarations, or other emergencies by providing strategies for effective acquisition planning and best practices agencies have developed in response to contracting during natural disasters and other emergencies.

Leading Practices for Lessons Learned

Our prior work has shown that the use of lessons learned—an approach of an organizational culture committed to continuous improvement—can increase communication and coordination. Collecting and sharing lessons learned—both positive and negative—allows agencies to communicate knowledge more effectively and to ensure that beneficial information is factored into planning, processes, and activities. This approach also provides a powerful method of sharing ideas for improving current and future operations. Collecting lessons learned throughout the course of an event, rather than just at the end, can help to ensure that lessons learned are captured as close as possible to the learning opportunity. Leading practices of a lessons learned process we and others identified include collecting, analyzing, validating, saving or archiving, and disseminating and sharing information and knowledge gained on positive and negative experiences.[31]

These leading practices generally build upon each other. For example, an organization with robust data collection methods is better able to gather enough information to effectively identify critical issues, analyze root causes, and develop recommendations. Further, an agency with a consistent, coordinated archiving mechanism, such as an electronic database, is better

---

[30] Executive Office of the President, Office of Management and Budget, Office of Federal Procurement Policy, *Emergency Acquisitions Guide* (January 2011).

[31] GAO-21-8, GAO-20-104, GAO-19-25, and GAO-12-901. Project Management Institute, Inc., *A Guide to the Project Management Body of Knowledge (PMBOK® Guide)* and *Implementing Organizational Project Management: A Practice Guide*. Center for Army Lessons Learned, *Establishing a Lessons Learned Program*.

able to demonstrate the leading practice for sharing lessons learned through access to such an archive.

Federal Agencies Obligated More Than $61 Billion on COVID-19-Related Contracts

As of May 31, 2021, federal agencies obligated about $61.4 billion in response to the COVID-19 pandemic. Most obligations (88 percent or $54.0 billion) were on contracts to vendors with prior federal contracting experience. Almost all vendors that received contract obligations in response to COVID-19 were registered in SAM at the time of award, and less than 1 percent of total COVID-19-related contract obligations went to vendors with documented records in FAPIIS, the repository for contractor performance and integrity information. Agencies cancelled or deobligated about 6 percent of the obligations for various reasons.[32]

Agencies Obligated Most COVID-19 Dollars to Vendors with Prior Federal Contracting Experience

As of May 31, 2021, federal agencies obligated about $61.4 billion in response to the COVID-19 pandemic. Most obligations (88 percent or $54.0 billion) were for contracts with vendors having prior federal contracting experience. Those vendors also accounted for 88 percent, or approximately 11,200, of the almost 12,800 vendors that received contract awards related to COVID-19. Although most contract obligations went to vendors with prior federal contracting experience, agencies awarded contracts to vendors without prior federal contracting experience at a higher percentage than they do in a typical year. In calendar year 2020, 16 percent of contracts awarded by agencies for the COVID-19 response were to vendors without prior federal contracting experience. In contrast, in the 5 most recent calendar years, between 2.7 to 3.8 percent of contracts were awarded to vendors without prior federal contracting experience.

Five agencies—DOD, HHS, USDA, the Department of Veterans Affairs, and DHS—accounted for the vast majority (89 percent) of the total COVID-

[32] A deobligation is a cancellation or reduction of previously incurred obligations.

19-related contract obligations. DOD had the highest obligations, accounting for 40 percent ($24.4 billion) of government-wide COVID-19- related contract obligations. The obligations by the top five agencies to vendors with prior federal contracting experience varied by agency. For example, DOD had the highest percentage of obligations to vendors with prior federal contracting experience, at 96 percent. USDA relied less on vendors with prior federal contracting experience, with only 64 percent of obligations going to such vendors. Figure 1 shows total obligations by agency, and the proportion of obligations going to vendors with or without prior federal contracting experience within each agency.

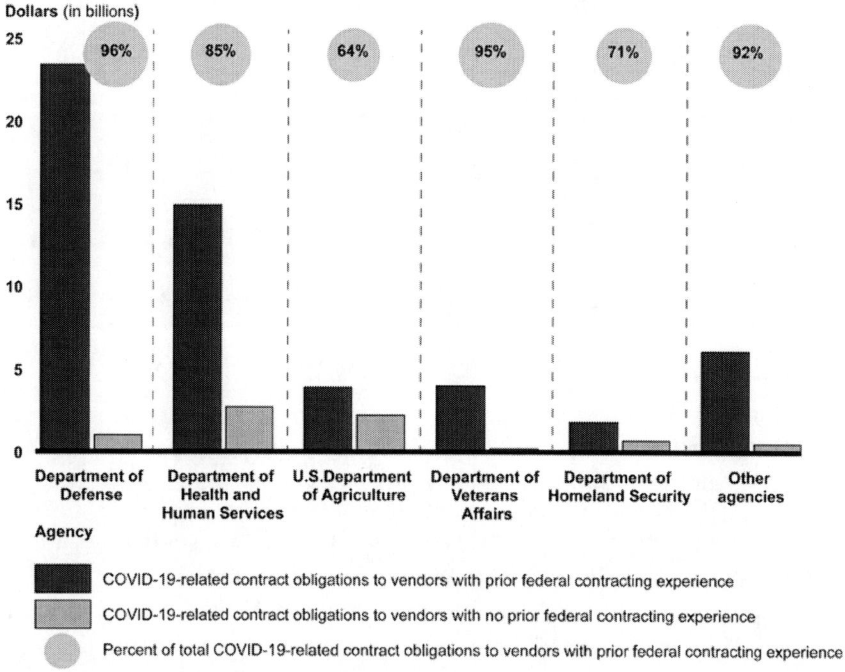

Source: GAO analysis of Fedefral Procurement Data System data. | GAO-21-528.

Figure 1. COVID-19-Related Contract Obligations and Proportion of Obligations to Vendors with Prior Federal Contracting Experience, by Federal Agency, as of May 31, 2021.

Contract obligations and the extent to which agencies relied on vendors with prior federal contracting experience also varied by the type of good or service. Government-wide, obligations on drugs and treatments, which include vaccines and therapeutics, were the highest of any good or service at

$14.3 billion, and 99 percent of these obligations were on contracts to vendors with prior federal contracting experience (see figure 2). The percentage of obligations to vendors with prior federal contracting experience, however, was lower for other goods or services. For example, of the $2.4 billion obligated for laboratory testing—which includes services related to diagnostic testing for COVID-19—48 percent of obligations were on contracts to vendors with prior federal contracting experience.

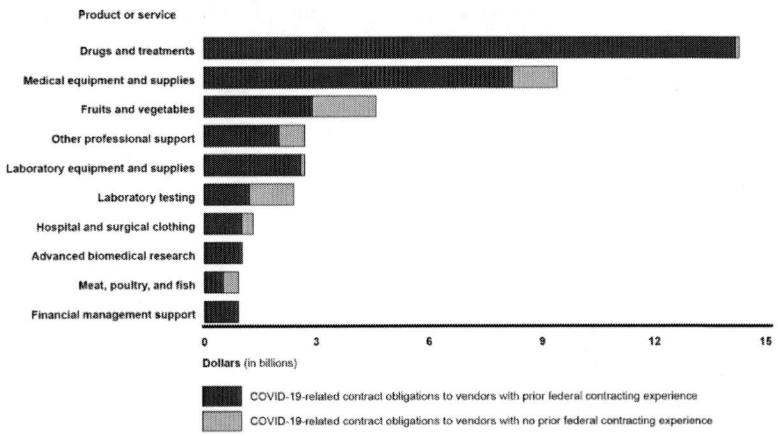

Source: GAO analysis of Federal Procurement Data System data. | GAO-21-528.

Figure 2. COVID-19-Related Contract Obligations and Proportion of Obligations to Vendors with Prior Federal Contracting Experience, by Top Goods and Services, as of May 31, 2021.

Agencies obligated a majority of COVID-19-related dollars to a small number of vendors. Seventy-one percent of obligations were for contracts awarded to 130 vendors, or 1 percent of the roughly 12,800 vendors receiving COVID-19-related contracts government-wide. Furthermore, as shown in figure 3, the top 10 vendors accounted for nearly one-third of the obligations.

Overall, agencies awarded contracts to over 8,100 small business vendors—nearly double the number of vendors awarded contracts that were not considered small businesses.[33] Small business vendors received 25 percent of the total COVID-19 contract obligations. Table 1 shows that a majority of small business vendors received less than $1 million in contract obligations.

[33] For the purposes of this report, a small business vendor is a vendor that was determined to be a small business for all of its COVID-19-related contract awards.

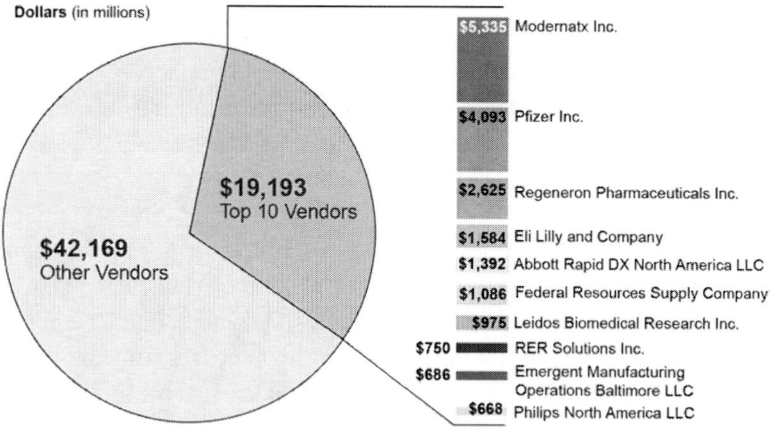

Source: GAO analysis of Federal Procurement Data System data. | GAO-21-528.

Figure 3. Government-wide COVID-19-Related Contract Obligations to Top 10 Vendors, as of May 31, 2021.

Table 1. COVID-19 Small Business Vendors by Obligation Range, as of May 31, 2021

Amount Obligated to Vendors (Obligation range in dollars)	Number of Small Business Vendors	Percent of Obligations to Small Business Vendors (within obligation range)
Over 1 billion	1	33
500 million-1 billion	1	10
100 million-499 million	14	14
10 million-99 million	169	30
1 million-9 million	719	47
Less than 1 million[a]	7,226	65
Total	8,130	25

Source: GAO analysis of Federal Procurement Data System data. I GAO-21-528.

[a] This includes vendors obligated zero or negative dollars due to cancelled contract obligations.

Almost All COVID-19 Vendors Were in the Government's Primary Contractor Registration System and Had No Prior Reports of Unsatisfactory Performance or Integrity

Almost all contract obligations in response to COVID-19 went to vendors registered in SAM at the time of award. Agencies have the flexibility to award contracts to vendors that are not registered in SAM during an emergency, among other circumstances, and 162 of the approximately 12,800 vendors receiving COVID-19-related contract obligations were not registered at the time of award, representing about 1 percent of the total number of vendors and of the $61 billion in total COVID-19 obligations.[34]

A small portion of COVID-19 contract obligations went to vendors with documented records in FAPIIS, the repository for contractor performance and integrity information.[35] Such vendors (119 in total) received about $507 million, less than 1 percent of total COVID-19-related contract obligations. HHS accounted for 52 percent of the $507 million, the Department of Veterans Affairs 24 percent, DOD 12 percent, and USDA 1 percent.[36] Contracting officers must document how the information in FAPIIS was considered when determining responsibility, and any action taken as a result of the information.

Agencies Cancelled $4 Billion in COVID-19- Related Contract Obligations

Approximately $4 billion, or 6 percent, of the COVID-19-related contract obligations were cancelled or deobligated, and these deobligations varied depending on the agency or good and service involved.[37] In some instances, agencies may modify a contract to deobligate funds to accommodate changes in the contract requirement, or to terminate a contract if a vendor does not fulfill the terms of the contract. For example, the federal government can partially or fully end a government contract before the contractor completes

[34] With certain exceptions—such as contracts awarded as responses to national emergencies—vendors must be registered in SAM at the time an offer or quotation is submitted to comply with annual representations and certifications requirements. FAR § 4.1102(a). For contracts awarded in emergency operations, the FAR provides that, if practical, contracting officers should modify the contract or agreement to require SAM registration. FAR § 4.1102(b).

[35] Documented records of unsatisfactory performance or integrity of a vendor in FAPIIS may include one or more of the following: criminal, civil, or administrative proceedings in connection with the award or performance of a government contract; terminations for default or cause; determinations of nonresponsibility because the vendor does not have a satisfactory performance record or a satisfactory record of integrity and business ethics.

[36] DHS accounted for 0.3 percent of obligations, which rounds to zero. Across the agencies, HHS awarded contracts to 19 vendors with documented records of unsatisfactory performance, the Department of Veterans Affairs to 37 vendors, DOD to 49 vendors, USDA to three vendors, and DHS to 11 vendors. Some vendors with unsatisfactory records of performance received COVID-19 contracts from multiple agencies.

[37] Agencies initially obligated $65 billion; however, $4 billion (6 percent) was cancelled. Given this, the net amount of total obligations was $61 billion.

performance by partially or fully terminating the contract. Depending on the circumstances, the government can terminate the contract either (1) for the convenience of the government or (2) for cause or default. A variety of factors can lead to the government's decision to terminate a contract. For example, when the government's requirements change, rendering continued performance unnecessary, the government may choose to terminate the contract for convenience. On the other hand, when a contractor fails or is anticipated to fail to perform its contractual obligations, the government may terminate the contract for default or, in the case of commercial item contracts, cause. DOD and HHS had the highest overall deobligations at $1.8 billion and $938 million, respectively. See figure 4 for a comparison of initial obligations and deobligations by agency.

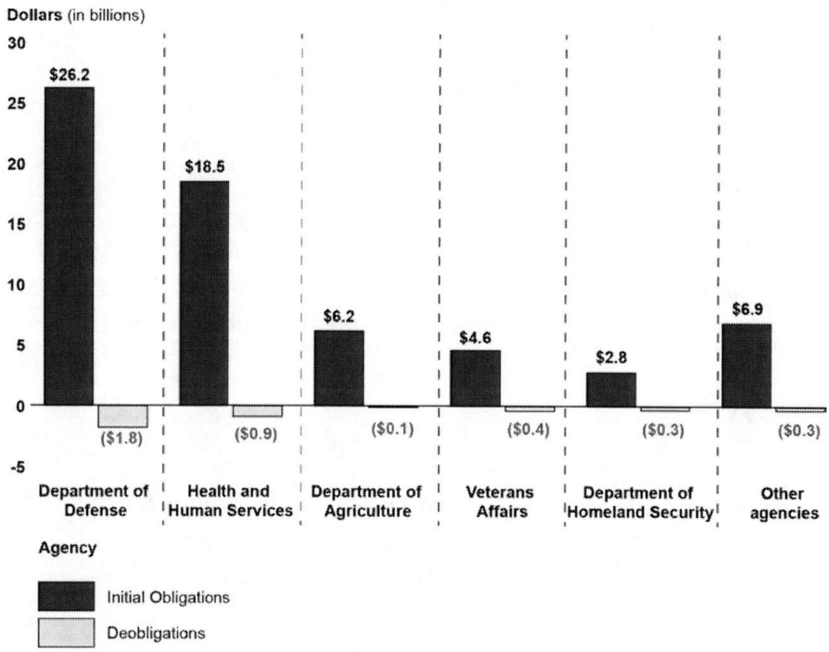

Source: GAO analysis of Federal Procurement Data System data. | GAO-21-528.

Figure 4. Initial COVID-19-Related Contract Obligations and Subsequent Deobligations, by Agency, as of May 31, 2021.

Our analysis of FPDS data identified a variety of reasons for agencies' deobligations. The majority of the approximately $4 billion in deobligations were coded as "Other Administrative Action." This code may be used due to, for example, a contract being modified to change the period of performance or decrease the requirements. Eleven percent of deobligations were due to contract terminations, with about one-third ($144 million) of these obligations related to contracts terminated for cause or default, and the other two-thirds ($276 million) related to contracts terminated for convenience. For example, some of the selected contracts we reviewed were terminated for cause after the vendor failed to deliver contracted medical supplies, such as N95 respirators. Other contracts we reviewed—such as contracts for ventilators or alternate care facilities—were terminated for convenience because the government no longer needed the good or service.

The percentage of contract deobligations varied by good or service. Generally, deobligations among the top goods and services were below 5 percent. For example, agencies deobligated about 1 percent, or $63 million, of initial obligations on fruits and vegetables. However, agencies deobligated about 13 percent, or $1.4 billion, of initial obligations on medical equipment and supplies—including personal protective equipment such as N95 respirators, isolation gowns, and medical gloves.

Government-wide there was little difference between deobligations on contracts to vendors with prior federal contracting experience compared to vendors without prior federal contracting experience. About $3.5 billion, or 6 percent, of the $57.4 billion in initial obligations to vendors with prior federal contracting experience was deobligated, compared to about $379 million, or 5 percent, of the $7.8 billion in initial obligations to vendors without prior federal contracting experience.

Contracting Officers Did Not Always Have Access to or Were Not Aware of Resources Available to Assess Prospective Vendors

Contracting officers rely on a variety of resources to assess prospective vendors. However, some agencies we reviewed did not have, or did not communicate to contracting officials, the resources available to assess prospective vendors during an emergency. Contracting officials we spoke with identified obstacles to assessing prospective vendors during the COVID-19 response. Further, available government-wide guidance provides limited information for assessing prospective vendors in an emergency.

Contracting Officials at Selected Agencies Used a Variety of Resources to Assess Prospective Vendors

We found that contracting officials at agencies across our four selected departments used a variety of resources to assess prospective vendors for our selected 28 contracts. These resources included government databases, private sector resources, assistance from other federal agencies, specific resources created by agencies in response to COVID- 19, and information identified by the contracting officers based on their own knowledge and experience. Figure 5 details examples of the resources that contracting officers responsible for our selected contracts said they used.

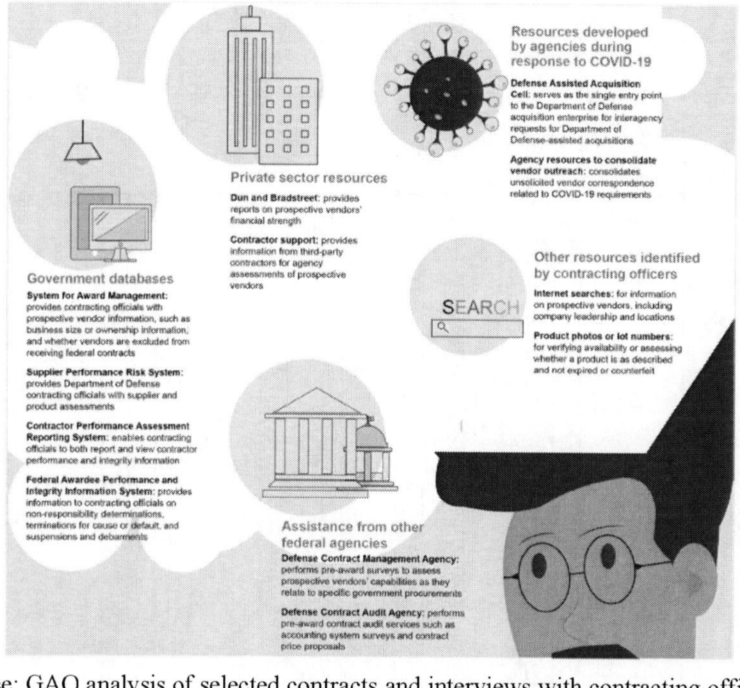

Source: GAO analysis of selected contracts and interviews with contracting officials. | GAO-21-528.

Figure 5. Examples of Resources Used by Contracting Officers to Assess Prospective Vendors for COVID-19-Related Contracts.

Overall, the number of contracting officers that used each of these resources across the contracts we selected varied. Table 2 provides details on how many of the 28 contracts leveraged each resource.

Table 2. Resources that Contracting Officials Identified Using to Assess Prospective Vendors Across Selected Contracts

Resource	Department of Defense (DOD)	Department of Health and Human Services (HHS)	U.S. Department of Agriculture (USDA)	Department of Homeland Security (DHS)
Government databases				
System for Award Management (prospective vendor business information)	7	6	7	7
Contractor Performance Assessment Reporting System (past performance information)	6	4	7	5
Federal Awardee Performance and Integrity Information System (past performance and integrity information)	7	5[d]	7	7
Supplier Performance Risk System (supplier and product assessments)[a]	2	N/A	N/A	N/A
Private sector information				
Dun and Bradstreet (financial strength information)	3	2	2	3
Third party contractor (additional information for vendor assessments)	0	2	0	0
Assistance from other federal agencies				
Defense Contract Management Agency (pre-award surveys)	2	0	0	1
Defense Contract Audit Agency (pre-award audit services)	3	0	0	0
Other resources				
Internet searches	0	4	0	1
Product photos[b]	0	0	0	2
Lot numbers[b]	0	1	0	0
Other resources[c]	1	2	0	1

Source: GAO analysis of selected contract files and interviews with contracting officials. | GAO-21-528. (Contracting officers used a variety of resources to assess prospective vendors across the seven contracts we selected at each agency.)

[a] The Supplier Performance Risk System is a DOD specific system, and therefore not applicable to contracts not awarded by DOD contracting officers.

[b] Product photos and lot numbers are not applicable to contracts for services.

[c] Other resources include support provided by the Defense Assisted Acquisition Cell and the White House.

[d] HHS officials were unable to locate documents to confirm whether they reviewed information in the Federal Awardee Performance and Integrity Information System for two of the selected contracts.

DOD and FEMA Have and Are Making Contracting Officers Aware of Resources for Assessing Prospective Vendors

Both DOD and FEMA have resources available to contracting officers to assist them in assessing prospective vendors. We found that contracting officers responsible for the DOD contracts we reviewed used resources the department had in place. We found limitations in the communication of available resources at FEMA; however, it is currently taking steps to update its guidance to better communicate the availability of these resources.

DOD Contracting Officers Used Agency-Specific Guidance to Assess Prospective Vendors

In relation to the seven contracts we reviewed at DOD, officials at DLA and the Department of the Army leveraged guidance and resources developed to support contracting officers' efforts to assess prospective vendors. For example:

- *DLA:* DLA's Defense Logistics Acquisition Directive instructs contracting officials to review the Defense Contractor Review List, which helps identify and communicate contractor performance, capability, and integrity issues for making a responsibility determination. The list contains treatment codes with recommended actions that contracting officials can take to mitigate risks. For example, the list includes codes that identify whether the contracting officer should consider requesting a pre-award survey for the vendor, whether the vendor has experienced financial difficulties that could jeopardize its ability to complete the contract, or whether the contracting official should request additional performance history information.[1] Contracting officers responsible for all three of the DLA COVID-19-related contracts we selected used the Defense Contractor Review List in their determinations of vendor responsibility, which some DLA contracting officials said allowed them to access notes and information from other DLA contracting officers' experiences working with a vendor.
- *Army:* In December 2019, the Department of the Army released guidance mandating use of the Contractor Responsibility

[1] Pre-award surveys can be used to evaluate a prospective contractor's capability, experience, and performance history.

Determination Bot. The bot is an automated tool that streamlines the process to collect responsibility information from government sources, including SAM and FAPIIS, allowing contracting officials to focus on making responsibility determinations more quickly and accurately by collecting relevant information into a memorandum that can be supplemented with additional vendor information. According to guidance issued by the Deputy Assistant Secretary of the Army for Procurement, the tool is intended to reduce the amount of time needed to make a responsibility determination, which is particularly important since contracting officers told us they operated under expedited time frames during the COVID-19 response. For the three Army contracts in our sample where use of the tool was required, contracting officials indicated they did so, allowing them to streamline the collection of required information to determine vendor responsibility.[2]

Additionally, USACE released further guidance and tools to assist contracting officers in assessing prospective vendors for their COVID- 19 alternate care facility missions. Specifically, based on work performed for these missions early in the pandemic, USACE developed a standardized set of 10 questions to include in solicitations to help provide contracting officers across USACE districts with key information to assess prospective vendors' abilities. USACE contracting officials we spoke with said that using the previously developed and approved solicitation questions allowed them to award contracts faster.

DHS Is in the Process of Better Communicating Its Resources to Assess Prospective Vendors

DHS and FEMA have developed several resources to assist contracting officers in assessing prospective vendors. For example:

- Following Hurricanes Harvey, Irma, and Maria in 2017—which occurred nearly back-to-back and affected nearly 47 million people

[2] For one of the three Army contracts in our sample, the contracting officer told us that they used the tool. However, the contracting officer has since left, and the agency was unable to provide supporting documentation. The fourth Army contract in our sample was awarded prior to the issuance of the December 2019 guidance requiring use of the tool for all Army contracts.

or 15 percent of the U.S. population—FEMA developed a disaster contract verification tool. The tool is a checklist to ensure contracting officers complete contracting steps, including documenting elements of responsibility, like satisfactory record of business ethics and integrity, and ability to comply with proposed delivery or performance schedules.

- In March 2020, FEMA also began requiring the use of a contractor assurance statement for prospective vendors to attest to their capabilities to perform a contract.
- In addition to FEMA's efforts, when the pandemic started, DHS Strategic Program Division officials explained that they vetted thousands of vendors offering goods and services, like personal protective equipment or other medical supplies, through interviews using a vendor vetting questionnaire. FEMA contracting officers also used the questionnaire to assess prospective vendors' capabilities.
- DHS developed a job aid to assist in responsibility determinations in November 2020. The job aid states that the responsibility determination is a first line of defense in determining whether a vendor can successfully meet the terms of a contract, and notes that this determination is especially important when a contracting officer is awarding a contract to a vendor that has no record of successful past performance or relevant prior experience. The aid identifies specific considerations for contracting officers related to responsibility factors identified in the FAR, and examples of additional evidence to request or collect if concerns arise when assessing a prospective vendor against those factors.

However, we found inconsistencies in how FEMA contracting officers used some resources for assessing prospective vendors. For example, contracting officials were instructed—by email and acquisition alert, respectively—to use the disaster contract verification tool and insert the contractor assurance statement in solicitations and contracts. Yet based on our review of the contract files and interviews with the responsible contracting officers, none of the officials responsible for the six selected contracts required to leverage the verification tool did so, and only three of six contracts in our sample contained the contractor assurance statement, as required.[3]

Based in part on our earlier findings following the 2017 hurricanes and wildfires, FEMA's contracting activity is taking steps to better communicate the resources available to contracting officers.[4] Specifically, FEMA contracting activity officials said that, as of May 2021, they are finalizing the FEMA Acquisition Manual, which will consolidate guidance and resources for contracting officers at the agency. Officials told us that the manual will include guidance for contracting officers to use the contractor assurance statement and the disaster contract verification tool, and that they are reviewing the agency's Disaster Contracting Desk Guide to ensure consistency on the use of these resources.

Contracting Officers at HHS Did Not Always Have Access to or Awareness of Resources Available to Assess Prospective Vendors

Contracting officials we spoke with at HHS's ASPR identified challenges with the time frames for awarding contracts and with working with new vendors in response to COVID-19. However, based on our review of seven selected contracts, we identified limitations in the resources available to ASPR contracting officials for assessing prospective vendors during the COVID-19 emergency and how information about those resources was communicated to contracting officers. *Standards for Internal Control in the Federal Government* state that management should use and internally communicate the necessary quality information to achieve the entity's objectives.[5]

---

[3] One of the selected contracts was awarded in 2017, prior to the development of the disaster contract verification tool and contractor assurance statement. FEMA issued task orders under this contract during the response to COVID-19.

[4] Our prior work found that FEMA lacked an updated strategy and guidance on its use of advance contracts. We recommended that FEMA update the strategy identified in its 2007 Advance Contracting of Goods and Services Report to Congress to clearly define the objectives of advance contracts, how they contribute to FEMA's disaster response operations, and whether and how they should be prioritized in relation to new post- disaster contract awards. We also recommended that FEMA update its Disaster Contracting Desk Guide to include guidance for whether and under what circumstances contracting officers should consider using advance contracts prior to making new post- disaster contract awards. FEMA agreed with our recommendations and identified the development of a FEMA Acquisition Manual as a mechanism to communicate FEMA- specific acquisition policies and processes to contracting personnel. FEMA has since taken other actions to address these recommendations. See GAO-19-93.

[5] GAO-14-704G.

We found that several contracting officers responsible for the contracts we reviewed either did not have access to or were not aware of resources that could have been used to assess prospective vendors awarded contracts in response to COVID-19. For example, contracting officials responsible for three of our seven selected contracts told us that they did not think they had access to Dun and Bradstreet credit reports.[6] Some of these contracting officials said that access to this service would have helped them to more thoroughly assess prospective vendors during their COVID-19 response efforts.[7]

Additionally, ASPR contracting officers were not always aware of available resources to help them assess financial capability. For example, a senior ASPR contracting official stated that ASPR has an audit evaluation team that contracting officers can use to conduct reviews of a prospective vendor's accounting system and financial capabilities.

However, contracting officers responsible for four of the seven contracts we selected were not aware of the types of assistance available from this team. Moreover, contracting officials responsible for one of our selected contracts determined that a prospective contractor had "necessary capacity and credit" to perform the contract, but could not cite any resources they used to assess whether the prospective vendor had adequate financial resources to perform the contract.[8]

Senior acquisition officials at ASPR told us that the resources available to contracting officers to determine responsibility were adequate, but that the agency had not reviewed the resources available to contracting officers to assess whether other resources could be useful. Yet as noted earlier, there was uncertainty among ASPR's contracting officers about what resources were available to them to assess prospective vendors, and the circumstances under which they should be used. These same senior ASPR officials added that they were not certain whether Dun and Bradstreet was still in use at federal agencies, and said the information available through Dun and Bradstreet was

---

[6] Dun and Bradstreet is a company that provides information on vendors' financial strength, among other things.

[7] A contracting officer within HHS's Biomedical Advanced Research and Development Authority (BARDA), which is housed within ASPR, stated that BARDA contracting officers may request Dun and Bradstreet reports for specific contracts, but that these are purchased on an ad hoc basis using purchase cards.

[8] Ultimately, the contract was terminated for cause after the vendor was unable to meet the required delivery schedule. We did not analyze whether there was any relationship between the contracting officer's determination regarding the contractor's "necessary capacity and credit" and the termination.

also available through SAM.gov. In fact, however, contracting officers at all of the other agencies we reviewed are using or requesting Dun and Bradstreet information as a resource to help them assess prospective vendors' financial capabilities, supplementing the information that vendors report in SAM.gov.

Further, a senior ASPR acquisition official noted that the audit evaluation team's services are not typically needed for contracts awarded through the Strategic National Stockpile. Officials told us that this is because stockpile officials are generally working with contractors with whom HHS has historically worked. However, ASPR, which has responsibility for the stockpile, accounted for about half, or $1.4 billion, of HHS's contract obligations for the COVID-19 response that went to vendors without prior federal contracting experience, and contracting officials associated with several of our selected contracts noted they were working with certain vendors for the first time. Without reviewing the resources that are available to contracting officers to assess prospective vendors to determine whether they are adequate and fully communicating the availability of such resources, ASPR increases the risk that its contracting staff will not have access to adequate resources to comprehensively assess prospective vendors during future emergencies.

In addition to lacking access to or awareness of resources to assess prospective vendors, several ASPR contracting officers we spoke with said they also did not have any ASPR-specific guidance or training they could leverage when assessing prospective vendors in an emergency. Contracting officers associated with two of our selected contracts noted the lack of ASPR-specific guidance as a challenge during the response. Moreover, contracting officers associated with several of our selected contracts said they relied on their experiences or guidance from working with other agencies—such as FEMA and the Centers for Disease Control and Prevention—to assess prospective vendors during the response to COVID-19.

Our prior work on the COVID-19 response effort has identified similar contracting issues related to ASPR's training and guidance for the use of Defense Production Act authorities—which can allow agencies to mitigate supply chain issues during an emergency. In November 2020, we reported that HHS planned to issue additional training and guidance on using Defense Production Act authorities to priority rate contracts, and that only three of 20 contracting officers had prior experience using the authority.[9] These challenges were also noted in a 2019 after-action report HHS conducted

[9] GAO-21-108.

following an emergency exercise on the nation's ability to respond to a large-scale outbreak of a novel virus. Further, in July 2021 we reported that ASPR did not have documented policies and procedures, including control and monitoring activities, related to its direct shipment procurement process.[10]

While ASPR has some acquisition guidance in place related to, for example, unsolicited proposals and ratification of unauthorized commitments, a majority of the policies ASPR officials identified as relevant to their emergency acquisition practices are still being developed or undergoing review. Further, while ASPR officials said they anticipate identifying additional policies based on the response to COVID-19, ASPR officials did not state that they plan to develop policies related to contracting or assessing prospective vendors during emergencies. Senior ASPR officials also noted that they did not think additional guidance related to assessing prospective contractors was necessary because contracting officials know what resources to look at when assessing prospective vendors based on the FAR. However, as we found, contracting officials were not always aware of available resources.

Moreover, we found that the Health and Human Services Acquisition Regulation only addresses responsibility determinations as they relate to certain procurements made by Indian Health Services. As noted earlier, contracting officers at other agencies within DOD and DHS have benefited from specific guidance on resources to assess prospective vendors, particularly when awarding contracts to vendors without successful past performance or prior relevant experience.

Standards for Internal Control in the Federal Government state that management should identify, analyze, and respond to risks related to achieving their objectives.[11] ASPR's stated mission is to save lives and protect Americans from 21st century health security threats and to lead the nation's medical and public health preparedness for, response to, and recovery from disasters and public health emergencies. Without internal guidance on practices for assessing prospective vendors, particularly during an emergency,

---

[10] GAO-21-551. ASPR used the direct shipment procurement process in response to COVID-19 to expedite delivery of medical supplies during the pandemic by allowing vendors to directly ship supplies to state, local, and territorial governments rather than shipping supplies directly to replenish the Strategic National Stockpile. We recommended that the Assistant Secretary for Preparedness and Response should update the policies and procedures, including related control and monitoring activities, for the Strategic National Stockpile to document the direct shipment procurement process and payment integrity risks. HHS did not concur with the recommendation.

[11] GAO-14-704G.

ASPR contracting officials are at risk of not being aware of the information available to help them more effectively perform their responsibilities.

USDA Developed a Checklist to Help Assess Vendors but Does Not Plan to Finalize It

USDA's AMS developed a draft responsibility checklist for emergency acquisitions to assist contracting officers in assessing prospective vendors, but does not plan to formalize or distribute it. AMS contracting officials used elements of the checklist to develop the solicitation for the Farmers to Families Food Box Program. Specifically, a contracting officer in AMS's Commodity Procurement Program responsible for awards in support of the Farmers to Families Food Box Program said the checklist was developed for emergency acquisitions to identify information that contracting officers should reference or request from prospective vendors to make a responsibility determination. The contracting officer said that incorporating elements of the checklist into the solicitation for the Farmers to Families Food Box Program—which was the solicitation for the seven contracts we selected—ensured that vendors' proposals would explicitly address certain elements of responsibility.

Additionally, for purposes of evaluating the offers submitted in connection with the Farmers to Families Food Box Program, AMS developed a step- by-step guide and an evaluation rubric, and provided training to technical evaluators on how to consistently assess prospective vendors for the program. According to AMS officials, they designed these new processes at the outset of the Farmers to Families Food Box Program to streamline the procurement process. Further, officials told us that these processes differed from their regular contracting activities for commodity procurement, which typically rely on a qualified bidders list.[12]

AMS officials said that they will maintain some of the tools, such as the evaluation rubric and step-by-step guide as reference materials, but that they do not anticipate the need to use them for future emergencies. AMS does not plan to formalize or distribute the draft responsibility checklist developed to assist contracting officers in assessing prospective vendors. Officials told us that AMS is not typically involved in emergency response activities, and said

[12] The FAR defines a qualified bidders list as a list of bidders who have had their products examined and tested and who have satisfied all applicable qualification requirements for that product or have otherwise satisfied all applicable qualification requirements. FAR § 9.201.

that the Farmers to Families Food Box Program was always intended to be a temporary program to address agricultural supply chain issues and increased joblessness during the COVID-19 response. Given these circumstances, officials did not provide the checklist as a tool to all AMS contracting officers, and officials said that it will not be formally adopted by the agency.

However, the official responsible for developing the checklist also said that the checklist was intended to help AMS award contracts during any declared emergency or disaster, not only during the COVID-19 response. Further, AMS officials told us they are in the process of determining next steps for future food distribution efforts following the additional $4 billion in funding for pandemic response USDA received as part of the American Rescue Plan Act of 2021 for purchasing and distributing food to individuals in need.[13]

Departmental guidance—such as the USDA contracting desk guide—addresses procedures for reporting determinations of non-responsibility but does not contain information to assist contracting officers in assessing prospective vendors. Additionally, AMS officials said they do not have any other regulations or guidance for contracting during emergencies.

According to a 2018 workforce analysis, AMS's Commodity Procurement Program previously identified the need to better align contracting processes across its branches, but staffing shortages and changes limited its efforts to do so.[14]

Standards for Internal Control in the Federal Government state that management should identify, analyze, and respond to risks related to achieving its objectives and should internally communicate necessary quality information, which would include contracting tools and guidance.[15] Although AMS is not typically involved in emergency response activities, not identifying and incorporating relevant contracting practices used to procure more than $6 billion worth of food into guidance puts the agency at risk of

---

[13] American Rescue Plan Act of 2021, Pub. L. No. 117-2, § 1001, 135 Stat. 4.

[14] GAO, *COVID-19: Sustained Federal Action Is Crucial as Pandemic Enters Its Second Year*, GAO-21-387 (Washington, D.C.: Mar. 31, 2021). In GAO-21-387, we identified challenges reporting contract obligations and managing contract documentation associated with USDA's Farmers to Families Food Box Program. We recommended, among other things, that the Administrator of AMS assess the contracting personnel needed to fully execute the award and administration of contracts in support of the Farmers to Families Food Box Program or successor future food distribution program, and take the necessary steps to ensure it has adequate contracting staff in place to award and administer any future contracts for the program. USDA neither agreed nor disagreed with our recommendation.

[15] GAO-14-704G.

losing the knowledge it has gained assessing vendors during an emergency, particularly as it considers future food distribution efforts.

Government-wide Emergency Acquisition Guidance Provides Limited Information on Resources for Assessing Prospective Vendors

OFPP's Emergency Acquisitions Guide outlines a number of management and operational best practices that agencies should consider when contracting during emergencies, but provides limited information on resources and practices agencies can use to assess prospective vendors prior to contract award.[16] In the course of our review, contracting officials identified obstacles to assessing prospective vendors during an emergency. Specifically, contracting officials cited urgent time frames and working with new vendors as factors that challenged their efforts to assess prospective vendors and that sometimes resulted in changes from their regular contracting processes. For example:

- *Urgent time frames*: AMS contracting officials told us that they had to operate under expedited time frames to award contracts, and that processes to assess vendors, such as determining responsibility and evaluating proposals, were sometimes conducted concurrently during the COVID-19 response rather than sequentially. Similarly, contracting officials at FEMA and ASPR said that under normal circumstances they would contact a prospective vendor's references to verify its performance information. However, officials said that they were unable to take this step because of the expedited time frames they were operating under during the COVID-19 response.
- *Working with new vendors*: A contracting officer from FEMA described challenges obtaining information on vendors providing goods or services during an emergency that differed significantly from the vendors' regular line of business. For example, the contracting officer noted this was the case when searching for information on a vendor that regularly provided furniture but began

[16] The OFFP guide is intended to supplement, not supplant, agency-specific guidance and the FAR. It is to be read in conjunction with parts 18 and 26 of the FAR, which address emergency acquisitions and other socioeconomic programs, respectively, and the National Response Framework documents published by FEMA.

> offering personal protective equipment at the beginning of the pandemic. Regarding the contract we selected, the contracting officer told us that given the market conditions for personal protective equipment at the beginning of the pandemic, they obtained the prospective vendor's business credit report—which the contracting officer said is not typical for procuring a commercial item or low dollar value contracts—to mitigate potential risks.

As previously mentioned, some agencies developed practices or resources to help address these obstacles, such as the Army's Contractor Responsibility Determination Bot and DHS's job aid for making responsibility determinations. Further, throughout the pandemic, OFPP officials explained that they maintained two websites—one publicly accessible and another strictly for government personnel—to convey COVID-19 acquisition related information, resources, and guidance.

OFPP's Emergency Acquisitions Guide also offers a number of resources and practices for agencies to consider during pre-emergency planning and in contract management and oversight during an emergency. These include identifying the products and services the agency required in previous emergencies, anticipating workforce needs before an emergency arises, adjusting internal processes to ensure flexibility during an emergency, and assessing emergency acquisitions following an emergency.

However, the OFPP guide does not include the practices or resources contracting officers can use to address obstacles they said they experienced related to assessing prospective vendors during COVID-19 or other recent emergencies. Specifically, the guide reiterates FAR requirements that contracts may only be awarded to responsible vendors and that such requirements are not waived during an emergency, but provides no additional guidance or best practices related to addressing potential obstacles contracting officers may encounter when assessing prospective vendors during an emergency. Furthermore, as previously discussed, not all agencies had or communicated resources available to contracting officers to assess prospective vendors during COVID-19, and some agencies that were involved in contracting for the COVID-19 response have not typically been involved in contracting in response to other recent disasters and emergencies, particularly AMS and ASPR.

Further, the Emergency Acquisitions Guide has not been updated since 2011, and, as of June 2021, several resources linked in the guide are no longer active or accessible. For example, the guide references a community of practice for emergency response—established by the Chief Acquisition Officers Council Emergency Response and Recovery Working Group—intended for agencies to share information about their policies and procedures, best practices, training resources, and other information of interest. However, OFPP staff told us the group is no longer operational. OFPP officials also stated that updates to the guide are driven by periodic discussions with senior procurement executives and by the rate of inquiries OFPP receives regarding emergency acquisitions, rather than on a regular schedule.

Our prior work following the 2017 hurricanes also identified other limitations in the available government-wide guidance on emergency acquisitions. In April 2019, we found that agencies experienced difficulty in determining whether a vendor resides or primarily does business in the local set-aside area after a disaster and recommended that OFPP provide clarifying information regarding contracting with local vendors after a disaster.[17] In May 2021, OFPP staff told us they plan to update the Emergency Acquisitions Guide to provide such clarifying information, but stated they could not provide a time frame for when the guide would be updated.

The intent of the Emergency Acquisitions Guide is to assist with planning and carrying out procurement activities during contingency operations, major disaster declarations, or other emergencies. *Standards for Internal Control in the Federal Government* state that management should use and externally communicate quality information that is current and accurate to achieve the entity's objectives on a timely basis.[18] The Emergency Acquisitions Guide does not account for obstacles contracting officers said they face when performing their responsibilities during an emergency, or more recent positive practices and resources that individual agencies have developed to address them. Without updating the Emergency Acquisitions Guide—including information on the resources and practices available to contracting officers to assess prospective vendors during an emergency—OFPP may miss the opportunity to provide agencies the information they need to mitigate the types of obstacles they faced during COVID-19 and other recent emergencies. Moreover, the lack of a regular process for updating the Emergency Acquisitions Guide leaves agencies, including those not typically involved in emergency response, without knowledge of the most current information on resources and practices they can use to mitigate obstacles during future emergencies.

---

[17] GAO-19-281.

[18] GAO-14-704G.

Table 3. Challenges and Outcomes Identified by Contracting Officials at the Departments of Defense (DOD), Health and Human Services (HHS), Agriculture (USDA) and Homeland Security (DHS)

Challenges	**DOD (DLA and Army)**	**HHS's ASPR**	**USDA's AMS**	**DHS's FEMA**	**Examples of Outcomes Highlighted by Officials**
Lack of contracting personnel in relation to volume of contract awards	-	X	X	-	ASPR officials said that as a result of limited contracting personnel, ASPR had to contract for support functions, like compiling contract file documentation. ASPR officials also said they relied heavily on interagency agreements with DOD and FEMA to procure goods and services and address contracting workforce shortfalls.
Working with vendors new to federal contracting or vendors supplying products they had not supplied before	X	X	X	X	DLA officials said that they often had to explain the federal contracting process—such as System for Award Management requirements or payment terms—when working with vendors that did not have prior federal experience, which can add time to the contracting process. A FEMA contracting official noted that one of the biggest challenges was determining whether vendors new to federal contracting or supplying a product for the first time were responsible and able to meet the delivery or performance terms of the contract.
Volume of communication from prospective vendors	X	X	X	X	FEMA officials said that the volume of prospective vendor communication they received was overwhelming and that contracting officials needed to work overtime to review vendor information, and in some cases it still delayed contract award.
Limited time frames and urgency to make contract awards	X	X	X	X	An AMS official said the speed with which contracts for the Farmers to Families Food Box Program were awarded and the sheer volume of awards affected contracting officials' ability to ensure accurate contract reporting and the compilation of complete contract files.[a]
Supply chain issues	X	X	-	X	According to DLA and ASPR officials, supply chain challenges related to the availability of supplies and raw materials and having to ship goods and materials from abroad led to delays in delivery and the ability to receive contracted goods.

Table 3. Continued

Challenges	DOD (DLA and Army)	HHS's ASPR	USDA's AMS	DHS's FEMA	Examples of Outcomes Highlighted by Officials
Contracting for supplies and services the agency does not typically buy	X	X	-	X	FEMA officials said they did not have expertise contracting for medical supplies, so were unfamiliar with some vendors and technical requirements for things like N95 respirators or gowns. As a result, officials said they relied heavily on technical expertise from DOD and HHS to determine whether vendor proposals met certain requirements.
Differing sources of contract requirements (e.g., other agencies, White House)	X	X	-	X	ASPR officials identified challenges receiving contract requirements from other agencies or the White House. For one selected contract, ASPR officials said that following changes in a White House requirement to deliver cloth masks to U.S. households, approximately 40 million masks are currently in storage at the Strategic National Stockpile or other locations. For two other selected contracts, ASPR contracting officials said that due to challenges with interagency communication about the number of ventilators needed for a contract, they ultimately had to partially terminate one of the contracts because not all of the ventilators ordered were needed.

Source: GAO summary of DLA, Army, ASPR, AMS, and FEMA information. I GAO-21-528.

Legend: DLA = Defense Logistics Agency Army = Department of the Army
ASPR = Office of the Assistant Secretary for Preparedness and Response
AMS = Agricultural Marketing Service
FEMA = Federal Emergency Management Agency
X = challenge identified by agency contracting officials
- = challenge not identified by agency contracting officials

[a] In March 2021, we reported that USDA faced data reporting and contract management challenges for its Farmers to Families Food Box Program. We recommended that USDA issue guidance to contracting officials on the use of the National Interest Action code for the Farmers to Families Food Box Program and assess the contracting personnel needed to fully execute the award and administration of existing contracts in support of the program or a successor food distribution program. USDA neither agreed nor disagreed with our recommendation. See GAO, *COVID-19: Sustained Federal Action Is Crucial as Pandemic Enters Its Second Year*, GAO-21-387 (Washington, D.C.: Mar. 31, 2021).

Agencies Identified Contracting Challenges and Positive Practices, but Shortfalls Exist in Lessons Learned Processes

Contracting officials from across our selected agencies identified a number of challenges and positive practices with contracting in response to COVID-19. While the agencies in our review are collecting and sharing lessons learned related to COVID-19, we identified shortfalls in these efforts, such as not including contracting personnel and contracting observations in lessons learned processes at some selected agencies and government-wide.

Agencies Identified Challenges and Positive Practices Related to Contracting Response to COVID-19

Contracting officials we spoke with in relation to the 28 contracts we reviewed identified a number of contracting challenges and positive practices that they experienced during the response to COVID-19. For example, contracting officials at DOD, HHS, and DHS said that the response to COVID-19 was unprecedented, and, as previously discussed, contracting officials at the agencies in our review stated that the limited time frames and urgency with which they had to assess prospective vendors and award contracts presented challenges. Table 3 describes challenges contracting officials identified across selected agencies, and the outcomes contracting officials associated with those challenges.

Officials also identified positive contracting practices that were established in response to COVID-19 or that assisted them in their ability to effectively respond during the pandemic.

- *Mechanisms to consolidate vendor communication:* Officials at DLA and USACE said they benefitted from their agencies establishing mechanisms to consolidate vendor communication about availability of goods and services. For example, officials at both agencies said they used centralized inboxes for vendors to communicate available goods and services. In some instances, these agencies "pre-vetted' vendors by asking for additional information on product availability, delivery terms, and pricing, before forwarding this information to contracting officials. According to USACE contracting officials, this vendor information was put into a repository that was accessible to their 43 districts, and having a list of available vendors helped them when performing market research.

- *Pre-existing contract vehicles*: Officials at DLA, USACE, ASPR, and FEMA were able to leverage some contracts that were awarded prior to the pandemic, which officials said allowed them to provide needed goods and services quicker. For example, following Hurricane Katrina in 2005, FEMA was required to establish advance contracts for goods and services typically needed following a disaster.[1] While FEMA's advance contracts are not specific to medical equipment and supplies, FEMA officials were able to leverage an advance contract for ambulance services during the response to COVID-19. The contracting officer associated with this contract said using the advance contract allowed the acquisition process to be streamlined, in part because the contractor was already vetted and familiar with the contract requirement and FEMA's processes. Similarly, following the H1N1 pandemic, the Biomedical Advanced Research and Development Authority (BARDA), within ASPR, awarded contracts to establish Centers for Innovation in Advanced Development and Manufacturing to support vaccine and other medical countermeasure manufacturing needs in support of future pandemics.[2] BARDA officials said that being able to leverage the already-established Centers allowed them to be responsive to COVID-19 vaccination needs during the pandemic.[3]

---

[1] Pub. L. No. 109-295, § 691 (codified at 6 U.S.C. § 791). We previously reported on challenges FEMA has faced using, managing, and coordinating advance contracts. See GAO-19-93.

[2] We previously reported on BARDA's efforts to establish Centers for Innovation in Advanced Development and Manufacturing. See GAO, *National Preparedness: HHS Has Funded Flexible Manufacturing Activities for Medical Countermeasures, but It Is Too Soon to Assess Their Effect*, GAO-14-329 (Washington, D.C.: Mar. 31, 2014).

[3] However, BARDA officials noted that limited funding for the Centers for Advanced Development and Manufacturing following the H1N1 pandemic posed challenges. Specifically, officials said that the Centers—operated by Texas A&M University Systems (which is one of our selected contracts) and Emergent Biosolutions (which was not one of our selected contracts)—faced staffing challenges due to limited funding that required them to quickly hire staff to support COVID-19 vaccine production. Recent Food and Drug Administration inspections at Emergent Biosolutions facilities responsible for COVID-19 vaccine production identified concerns related to cross-contamination of vaccine materials, the sanitation, size, and design of the facility, and staff adherence to process and production control procedures.

Agencies Are Collecting and Sharing COVID-19 Lessons Learned, but Some Agencies Have Not Included Contracting Issues

Agencies across the four selected departments in our review—DOD, HHS, USDA, and DHS—had in place or developed processes to collect and share lessons learned related to COVID-19, and these processes are ongoing or at various stages of completion. However, the lessons learned processes at HHS and DHS have not included contracting personnel or contracting observations.

- *DOD:* Within the Army and DLA, efforts to collect and share lessons learned in response to COVID-19 have been ongoing. For example, in addition to an "in-stride" review—completed while the alternate care facility mission was still ongoing in May 2020—USACE headquarters compiled a final after-action report on its COVID-19 response and alternate care facility mission in August 2020, which included after- action reports from across the districts and divisions. According to DLA officials, they collected acquisition lessons learned internally and completed a review of selected COVID-19 contracts to identify additional contracting lessons learned in May 2021.

  In addition to these component specific efforts, in December 2020, DOD's COVID-19 Task Force completed a strategic review of the department's response to COVID-19.[4] According to task force officials, they collected and analyzed over 2,000 observations from across the department, including reviewing component specific after- action reports, based on the department's existing guidance for the Chairman of the Joint Chiefs of Staff Joint Lessons Learned Program.[5] This analysis culminated in 84 recommendations related to DOD's organization, people, mission, and support to national and international response efforts. According to DOD officials, these recommendations have been archived and shared over the Joint Lessons Learned Information System. DOD COVID-19 Task Force

[4] DOD, *Strategic Review: The Department of Defense Response to the COVID-19 Pandemic* (December 2020). DOD's Strategic Review also included observations from other federal agencies on the actions DOD took in response to COVID-19, but the review states it was not intended to provide a detailed examination of the actions taken by the department's interagency partners in their response efforts.

[5] DOD, Chairman of the Joint Chiefs of Staff Instruction 3150.25G, *Joint Lessons Learned Program* (Jan. 31, 2018).

officials said they are still analyzing and validating lessons learned through the development of implementation and action plans for the recommendations, which they expect to complete in July 2021. DOD has also continued to gather observations to identify lessons learned as part of a Comprehensive Review focused on its COVID-19 response efforts through April 2021, which it anticipates completing in the fall of 2021.

- *HHS:* According to ASPR Exercise, Evaluation and After Actions (E2A2) officials, they are in the process of collecting data on the response to COVID-19 because the pandemic response is ongoing. The E2A2 division's lessons learned process uses after-action reports and a Corrective Action Program, aligned with DHS's Homeland Security Exercise and Evaluation Program, to collect, analyze, and report on observations following real world public health emergencies or exercises. To further improve HHS's ability to provide health and medical resources, corrective actions from real world public health emergencies and exercises generally become objectives in future training and exercises. E2A2 officials said that during and after a real world event or exercise, they send email surveys to all HHS personnel requesting input, and perform "hotwashes" with stakeholders to gather observations before consolidating the information based on trends and creating an after-action report.[6] Following the completion of the after-action report, observations and recommendations are resolved through the development of corrective actions that are then prioritized and tracked.
- *USDA:* AMS officials told us they do not have a formal process to collect lessons learned related to the Farmers to Families Food Box Program. However, USDA did conduct a preliminary review of its COVID-19-related commodity purchasing and distribution in January 2021, prior to issuing any new solicitations for the Farmers to Families Food Box Program, as required by the Consolidated Appropriations Act, 2021 (P.L. 116-260). The preliminary review identified observations and lessons learned from throughout the program and noted that USDA had been collecting, analyzing, and

[6] A "hotwash" is a facilitated discussion held immediately after an exercise or real world event among the individuals involved. It captures feedback about any issues, concerns, or proposed improvements that the individuals may have about the exercise or event.

addressing input on the program from participants, Congress, and the general public, as the program progressed. According to the preliminary review, USDA will analyze and apply lessons learned from the program to improve future commodity procurement efforts. Further, in April 2021, AMS officials told us that they have continued to collect input from both internal and external stakeholders and are working with a contractor to consolidate all of the input received and determine next steps with USDA leadership.

- *DHS:* FEMA's Continuous Improvement Program is responsible for collecting observations and conducting after-action reviews following a disaster. In the summer and fall of 2020, the Program provided preliminary briefings to FEMA leadership on selected after-action report focus areas. In January 2021, the Continuous Improvement Program completed its Initial Assessment Report of FEMA's COVID- 19 Operations from January 2020 through September 2020.[7] FEMA conducted its assessment by gathering data from across the agency using interviews, surveys, and "hotwashes," and analyzing and validating findings. The initial assessment included 32 findings and 57 recommendations related to coordinating structures and policy; resources; supporting state, local, tribal, and territorial governments; preparedness and information analysis; and organizational resilience. According to FEMA Continuous Improvement Program officials, these observations have been entered into the issue resolution system for tracking and shared in a database available to all FEMA employees.

DOD's and USDA AMS's lessons learned processes in response to COVID-19 have included contracting officials and their observations, but HHS ASPR's and DHS FEMA's formal lessons learned processes have not, posing the risk that contracting challenges and positive practices will not be appropriately analyzed, validated, archived, and shared to inform future efforts.

- *DOD:* Both USACE and DLA have captured contracting lessons learned related to their COVID-19 response missions. USACE's "in-stride" and final after-action report from its alternate care facility

[7] FEMA, Pandemic Response to Coronavirus Disease 2019 (COVID-19): Initial Assessment Report, FEMA Operations January through September 2020 (January 2021).

mission included contracting lessons learned, such as developing and communicating sample documents and templates, establishing lists of emergency contractors, and promoting internal and external communication. Following a review of contracts awarded in response to COVID-19, in May 2021, DLA reported on contracting lessons learned, such as establishing a group of contingency contracting officers able to support future emergency response efforts, and continuing to use a team that was established to assess prospective vendors. More broadly, as part of DOD's Strategic Review, DOD COVID-19 Task Force officials said they included input from contracting officials as part of their data collection efforts, and we found that the review highlights findings and recommendations related to DOD's establishment of the Joint Acquisition Task Force and extensive acquisition support to other agencies, like HHS. According to a DOD COVID-19 Task Force official, contracting lessons learned continue to be gathered as part of the department's Comprehensive Review.

- *USDA:* While less formal, AMS has also collected internal and external feedback on the program, and identified and applied contracting lessons learned to achieve the program's goals throughout the Farmers to Families Food Box Program. For example, based on information collected following initial awards made for the program, AMS streamlined its contracting process by using basic ordering agreements, which officials said provided AMS with greater flexibility to specify requirements as the program progressed.[8] Further, under the basic ordering agreement solicitation, AMS refined requirements related to the content and quantities of boxes to be delivered, and required additional documentation related to subcontractor agreements to ensure that vendors were fully accounting for the costs of delivering food boxes to their final destination instead of a distribution center.
- *HHS:* ASPR's E2A2 division is still in the process of formally collecting lessons learned from the response to COVID-19, but in February 2021, officials told us they do not plan to include contracting officials or lessons learned in their efforts. ASPR

[8] For subsequent contract awards under the Farmers to Families Food Box Program, AMS officials established basic ordering agreements with vendors, which then competed amongst themselves to fulfill specific requirements for the program.

contracting officials we spoke with identified challenges and lessons learned from the response to COVID-19, and, for most of the contracts in our review, contracting officials said they had communicated these challenges and lessons learned informally to their branch leadership or to the ASPR Head of Contracting Activity. According to senior ASPR contracting officials, there have been informal discussions about challenges and lessons learned in response to COVID-19 during monthly meetings with contracting leadership, and these lessons learned have been communicated to the Office of Acquisitions—which is responsible for providing departmental leadership for acquisition functions within the Office of the Assistant Secretary for Financial Resources. In February 2021, the Office of Acquisitions compiled preliminary contracting lessons learned from ASPR and other HHS component contracting activities. As of April 2021, contracting officials within ASPR and the Office of Acquisitions said they were determining next steps related to implementing the lessons learned they had identified. However, these officials said that they had not received any communication from E2A2 officials about sharing contracting lessons learned or provided lessons learned through the email surveys E2A2 sends to solicit feedback. Several ASPR contracting officials we spoke with during our review emphasized the importance of collecting contracting lessons learned.

- According to E2A2 officials, contracting has not been identified as a shortfall or priority for reporting by HHS leadership, and E2A2 has not received contracting input. However, we found that preliminary contracting lessons learned identified by the Office of Acquisitions and ASPR contracting officials are related to the topics E2A2 identified for inclusion in its planned after-action reports. For example, ASPR contracting officials told us that they did not have to award new contracts to support the mission to repatriate U.S. citizens from abroad early in the response to COVID-19 because they already had pre-existing contracts in place to provide all of the necessary services and medical support. Further, the Office of Acquisitions identified cross-agency contracting collaboration and confusion about agencies' responsibilities acquiring goods and services to protect the public against COVID-19. That office recommended establishing memorandums of understanding with other agencies involved in the response. E2A2 officials said they are issuing an after-action report focused on the repatriation mission and plan to issue an after-action report on interagency coordination, but contracting practices and lessons learned related to these areas have not been provided or included.[9]

- *DHS:* While FEMA's Continuous Improvement Program has a formal process for collecting, analyzing, validating, and archiving lessons learned, its initial assessment on the response to COVID-19 does not include contracting lessons. According to an official within FEMA's contracting activity, FEMA established community of practice listening sessions in April 2020 to promote training and educational opportunities and identify challenges and best practices for knowledge sharing. The official stated that these listening sessions are intended to inform the topics covered in the annual disaster webinar that they provide to contracting officials. However, as of April 2021, senior FEMA procurement officials told us they had not collected challenges or lessons learned from contracting officials. Further, officials with five of the seven contracts we reviewed said they had not communicated their lessons learned within the agency, and our review of the lessons learned identified in FEMA's May 2021 annual disaster webinar were specific to their regional offices and not FEMA headquarters contracting personnel.

  An official from FEMA's Continuous Improvement Program said they interviewed FEMA's Head of Contracting Activity and Deputy Head of Contracting Activity as part of their initial assessment on the response to COVID-19. The Continuous Improvement Program official said contracting was not a priority issue at that time, and procurement challenges and lessons learned did not align with broader themes identified in their data collection efforts and so were not included in their reporting. However, some of the challenges and positive practices FEMA contracting officials identified to us are related to findings in FEMA's initial assessment. For example, FEMA contracting officials noted that having DOD support the

---

[9] We previously reported that ASPR has not obtained input from key stakeholders— specifically other emergency support function agencies and territorial governments—as part of its after-action reporting following the 2017 hurricanes. We recommended that ASPR take steps to ensure that key external parties are incorporated in the development of HHS's after action reports. HHS officials agreed with the recommendation and as of May 2021, HHS's efforts to incorporate key external parties in after-action reports were ongoing. See GAO, *Disaster Response: HHS Should Address Deficiencies Highlighted by Recent Hurricanes in the U.S. Virgin Islands and Puerto Rico,* GAO-19-592 (Washington, D.C.: Sept. 20, 2019).

> technical evaluation of vendor proposals for medical supplies was helpful, since FEMA does not have expertise purchasing medical supplies. FEMA contracting officials also described significant challenges managing vendor communication about available goods and services and contracting in an environment where the availability of medical supplies was limited. FEMA's initial assessment on its response to COVID-19 includes findings related to interagency coordination structures, scarcity of medical supplies, and consistency of private sector engagement, but these findings did not include specific perspectives from contracting officials on their challenges and best practices.

Leading practices of a lessons learned process we and others have identified include collecting, analyzing, validating, archiving, and sharing information and knowledge on positive and negative experiences.[10] Further, The Standard for Program Management, produced by the Program Management Institute, Inc., states that program managers should actively engage key stakeholders throughout the life cycle of the program, which would include contracting officials responsible for awarding contracts worth billions of dollars for needed goods and services to respond to the pandemic.[11] The response to COVID-19 has been unprecedented and differed from other disasters and emergencies, as it affected the entire country and world rather than just one state or region. In addition, the response to the pandemic is currently in its second year, compared to typical emergency response efforts that can often be measured in weeks. Without taking steps to collect, analyze, and validate contracting lessons learned more than a year into the response, ASPR and FEMA—agencies that account for 20 percent of the $61 billion in contract obligations made in response to COVID-19—are at risk of not being able to apply and share critical contracting lessons learned related to the pandemic that could inform ongoing and future emergency response efforts.

---

[10] GAO-21-8, GAO-20-104, GAO-19-25, and GAO-12-901. Project Management Institute, Inc., *A Guide to the Project Management Body of Knowledge (PMBOK® Guide)* and *Implementing Organizational Project Management: A Practice Guide*. Center for Army Lessons Learned, *Establishing a Lessons Learned Program.*

[11] Program Management Institute, Inc. *The Standard for Program Management,* Fourth Edition (2017).

Contracting Officials Were Not Always Aware of or Involved in Collecting or Sharing Interagency Lessons Learned

Contracting officials we spoke with identified extensive interagency coordination related to contracting during the response to pandemic, but they were not always aware of or involved in interagency lessons learned processes. For example, as noted earlier, HHS established memorandums of understanding with DOD and FEMA for those agencies to provide contracting services and support for the acquisition of medical supplies and services. ASPR officials noted that these memorandums of understanding were essential because they did not have sufficient contracting workforce to meet their steady state mission, let alone the response to COVID-19. FEMA and DOD contracting officials also noted that they relied on technical support and expertise from various HHS components, particularly when awarding contracts for medical supplies and services that they do not typically purchase.

Moreover, according to contracting officials, 20 of the 21 contracts in our review awarded by DLA, the Department of the Army, FEMA, and ASPR involved interagency coordination related to the development of the requirement, assessment of prospective vendors, or contract administration efforts.[12] Figure 6 provides examples of the variety of government entities that were involved in identifying requirements, providing information in support of or performing vendor assessments, or contract administration efforts for these selected contracts.

Although interagency coordination has been critical to the response, contracting officials we spoke with at DOD, HHS, and DHS were not consistently aware of or involved in formal interagency lessons learned collection or reporting. Officials at DOD, HHS, and DHS identified some methods for communicating interagency lessons learned internally. For example, DOD's USACE officials said that in coordination with HHS, they identified areas to improve or sustain related to their alternate care facility mission, which included contracting. According to DLA officials, they have coordinated with the Defense Threat Reduction Agency, other DOD entities, FEMA, and HHS to capture lessons learned and best practices, including those related to contracting, from the COVID-19 response as part of an Interagency Lessons Learned Task Force. However, senior contracting officials at ASPR,

[12] The other seven contracts we selected for review were from USDA. Given the nature of those contracts, which were for food distribution efforts under the Farmers to Families Food Box Program, AMS officials said these contracts did not involve interagency coordination.

FEMA, and USACE said they were not aware of and had not participated in this or any other formal efforts to capture contracting lessons learned across the three agencies.

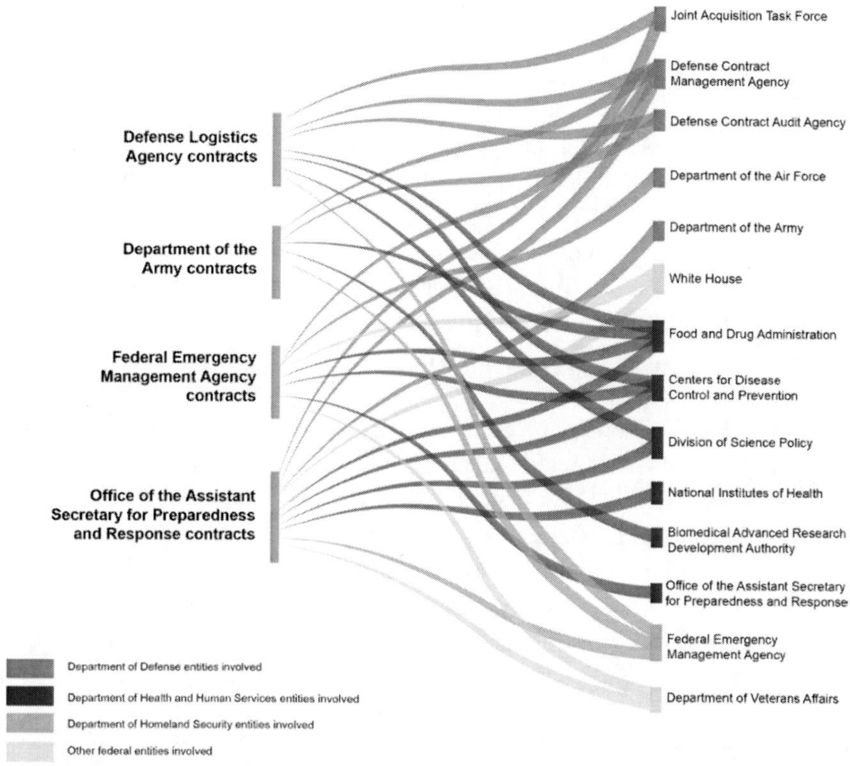

Source: GAO analysis of Department of Defense, Department of Health and Human Services and Department of Homeland Security information and interviews with contracting officials. | GAO-21-528.

Note: Lines from selected agency contracts to various government entities indicate those entities involvement in identifying contract requirements, providing information in support of or performing vendor assessments related to the contract, or contract administration efforts.

Figure 6. Examples of Interagency Contracting Coordination across Selected Contracts.

Further, agency officials responsible for gathering and reporting on lessons learned told us they have been focusing on their own agency lessons learned instead of coordinating with other agencies to identify interagency lessons learned. For example, while both FEMA's and DOD's after-action reports included challenges related to interagency coordination, both reports state that they are focused on the actions of their respective agencies versus collecting interagency lessons learned. During the course of our review, FEMA Continuous Improvement Program officials told us they have not shared information on challenges, positive practices, or lessons learned with other agencies, beyond some informal communication with officials within ASPR.[13] A FEMA Continuous Improvement Program official further noted that there is no policy identifying responsibilities for conducting interagency after-action reports. E2A2 division officials within HHS told us that information sharing among agencies has been a challenge, and that, while there had been some informal interagency coordination among FEMA and DOD, none of the agencies want to tell the others what did not go well.

According to a DOD COVID-19 Task Force official, the Homeland Preparedness Response Interagency Policy Committee—which replaced the Domestic Resilience Group Interagency Policy Committee on the National Security Council—is expected to lead efforts for a government-wide COVID-19 after-action report.[14] As of April 2021, the Task Force official said that group's charter was still being finalized, and the Exercise and Evaluation sub-Interagency Policy Committee that would lead such an effort has not yet been established. According to an HHS E2A2 official, DOD, HHS, and DHS are represented on this sub-Interagency Policy Committee, and it would be an appropriate interagency body for identifying and sharing lessons learned in any response.

Further, interagency lessons learned may also be collected by the Emergency Support Function Leadership Group—a body of senior officials from each of the emergency support functions tasked with coordinating responsibilities and resolving operational and preparedness issues related to interagency response activities. However, according to officials, as of April 2021, no corrective actions or lessons learned for COVID-19 contracting, or more broadly, had been identified. Emergency Support Function Leadership Group officials said that they rely on federal agencies that lead the Emergency Support Functions to identify corrective actions and that, while contracting lessons learned may be identified at some point, there are currently no efforts

---

[13] Towards the end of our review, a FEMA Continuous Improvement Program official stated that FEMA's initial assessment report is publicly available for other agencies to review.

[14] The National Security Council's Domestic Resilience Group was a policy group charged with discussing the authorities, policies, capabilities, and structures in place for a domestic response.

underway to take action on agency after-action recommendations because the response to COVID- 19 is ongoing.[15]

Leading practices of a lessons learned process we and others have identified include collecting, analyzing, validating, archiving, and sharing information and knowledge on positive and negative experiences.[16] The Center for Army Lessons Learned handbook on Establishing a Lessons Learned Program—which is intended to assist any government or civilian organization that wants to develop a lessons learned capability—notes that performing lessons learned practices throughout the course of an event, rather than just at the end, can help to ensure that lessons learned are captured as close to the learning opportunity as possible.[17] Further, key practices to enhance and sustain collaboration state that, in order for agencies to identify areas where collaboration could improve, they need to monitor, evaluate, and report the results of collaborative efforts—such as those related to interagency contracting during an emergency—to key decision makers.[18] Without efforts to ensure that key agencies involved in the response to COVID-19 are collecting and sharing interagency contracting lessons learned, federal agencies involved in the response are at risk of missing an opportunity to memorialize contracting and coordination practices that were successful, as well as those that were not, for future emergencies.

---

[15] Our prior work found that some emergency support function agencies—such as USACE and the Coast Guard—did not have formal processes to solicit and share input from officials involved in emergency response efforts to the Emergency Support Functions Leadership Group. We recommended that USACE and the Coast Guard establish formal processes to solicit input from officials involved in the agency's response and recovery efforts, and share that input with the Emergency Support Function Leadership Group.
Both agencies agreed with the recommendations, and in July 2020, USACE revised its Response to All Hazards Events Plan with steps to communicate lessons learned following a disaster to the group. As of April 2021, the Coast Guard's efforts to update its After-Action Report Policy were still ongoing. GAO-19-281.

[16] GAO-21-8, GAO-20-104, GAO-19-25, and GAO-12-901. Project Management Institute, Inc., *A Guide to the Project Management Body of Knowledge (PMBOK® Guide)* and *Implementing Organizational Project Management: A Practice Guide*. Center for Army Lessons Learned, *Establishing a Lessons Learned Program.*

[17] Center for Army Lessons Learned, *Establishing a Lessons Learned Program.*

[18] GAO, *Results-Oriented Government: Practices That Can Help Enhance and Sustain Collaboration among Federal Agencies*, GAO-06-15 (Washington, D.C.: Oct. 21, 2005).

Conclusion

Federal contracts played a critical role in meeting the unprecedented demand for billions of dollars in goods and services in response to COVID-19. Contracting during an emergency can pose a unique set of challenges as officials face a significant amount of pressure to provide goods and services as quickly as possible under difficult market conditions. To help contracting officers perform assessments of prospective vendors under these conditions during COVID-19, some agencies used or developed resources or guidance to supplement what is required by federal regulation. However, reviewing and communicating available resources for assessing prospective vendors and providing additional guidance for contracting during emergencies could improve ASPR contracting officers' ability to perform their responsibilities under tight time frames during ongoing and future emergencies. Additionally, identifying and incorporating relevant contracting experiences from its response to COVID-19 could improve AMS's food distribution efforts now and in the future. Further, updating OFPP's government-wide guidance to reflect the resources agencies have relied on to mitigate obstacles of assessing prospective vendors in recent emergencies, and establishing a process for regular updates to the guidance, will ensure that all federal agencies can benefit from these practices during future emergency response efforts.

In addition to improvements in communicating resources and guidance for assessing prospective vendors, agencies' experiences contracting in response to COVID-19 provide an important opportunity to capture and share lessons learned. Agencies identified a number of challenges and positive practices when contracting in response to COVID-19, but without established mechanisms to formally collect and share lessons learned from stakeholders involved with contracting at ASPR and FEMA, these agencies will be unable to apply lessons learned and positive processes to their ongoing pandemic response or future emergencies. Moreover, given the significant role that interagency contracting and coordination played in agencies' efforts to procure needed goods and services, effective coordination and communication among key emergency support function agencies is critical to ensure that interagency contracting lessons learned are memorialized in a timely manner.

Recommendations for Executive Action

We are making a total of 10 recommendations, including four to HHS, one to USDA, one to FEMA, two to OFPP, one to DOD, and one to DHS.

The Secretary of Health and Human Services should direct the Assistant Secretary for Preparedness and Response to review and fully communicate the resources available to contracting officers for assessing prospective vendors—including resources to assess financial capability. (Recommendation 1)

The Secretary of Health and Human Services should direct the Assistant Secretary for Preparedness and Response to develop internal guidance that includes information for contracting officers related to contracting and assessing prospective vendors during emergencies. (Recommendation 2)

The Secretary of Agriculture should direct the Administrator of the Agricultural Marketing Service to evaluate the contracting practices established to assess vendors and implement the Farmers to Families Food Box Program to determine what practices could be used for future emergency procurements and incorporate those practices into internal guidance. (Recommendation 3)

The Administrator of the Office of Federal Procurement Policy should revise the Emergency Acquisitions Guide, based on outreach to agencies involved in the COVID-19 response, to account for information on the obstacles contracting officers may face when assessing prospective vendors during an emergency and key practices or resources to address those obstacles, and communicate those revisions to agencies once complete. (Recommendation 4)

The Administrator of the Office of Federal Procurement Policy should establish a process and time frames for regularly updating the Emergency Acquisitions Guide to ensure resources and practices federal agencies can use when contracting during an emergency are current. (Recommendation 5)

The Secretary of Health and Human Services should ensure that, as part of the Exercise, Evaluation and After Actions Division's ongoing after- action reporting and corrective action program, contracting lessons learned in response to COVID-19 and future emergency response efforts are collected, analyzed, validated, archived, and shared to inform HHS's contracting efforts in response to ongoing and future emergencies. (Recommendation 6)

The Administrator of the Federal Emergency Management Agency should direct the Head of Contracting Activity to establish a formal process to (1) collect contracting lessons learned from COVID-19 and future emergency response efforts; and (2) ensure contracting lessons learned are shared with the Continuous Improvement Program for inclusion in FEMA's formal lessons learned process to inform FEMA's contracting efforts in response to ongoing and future emergencies. (Recommendation 7)

The Secretary of Defense, in coordination with the Secretaries of Homeland Security and Health and Human Services, should ensure that input from contracting officials on interagency contracting lessons learned in response to COVID-19 is collected and shared as part of government- wide efforts to collect, analyze, and report on lessons learned. (Recommendation 8)

The Secretary of Health and Human Services, in coordination with the Secretaries of Defense and Homeland Security, should ensure that input from contracting officials on interagency contracting lessons learned in response to COVID-19 is collected and shared as part of government- wide efforts to collect, analyze, and report on lessons learned. (Recommendation 9)

The Secretary of Homeland Security, in coordination with the Secretaries of Defense and Health and Human Services, should ensure that input from contracting officials on interagency contracting lessons learned in response to COVID-19 is collected and shared as part of government- wide efforts to collect, analyze, and report on lessons learned. (Recommendation 10)

Agency Comments

We provided a draft of this report to DOD, HHS, USDA, the Department of Veterans Affairs, DHS, and the Office of Management and Budget (OMB) for review and comment. DOD, HHS, and DHS provided written comments, which are reproduced in appendices II, III, and IV, and USDA and OMB responded via email. Collectively, the agencies concurred with 9 of the 10 recommendations. DHS also provided technical comments, which we incorporated as appropriate. DOD, HHS, USDA, OMB, and the Department of Veterans Affairs had no technical comments on the draft report.

DOD, HHS, DHS, and USDA concurred with the recommendations made to each of their agencies and generally identified steps they plan to take to address them. In its concurrence with our seventh recommendation, FEMA requested that we consider the recommendation resolved and close as implemented based on actions it had previously taken. In DHS's written comments, FEMA cited actions, such as interviews with FEMA's Head and Deputy Head of Contracting Activity and other efforts by FEMA to identify challenges and promote knowledge sharing through listening sessions. These efforts are, in general, already referenced in our report. Furthermore, we found that contracting officials involved with most of the FEMA contracts in our review had not communicated their lessons learned related to contracting during COVID-19 within the agency.

Moreover, several of the contracting officials we spoke with said they were not aware of any efforts to collect lessons learned and had not been asked to provide any, raising concerns about the efficacy of FEMA's Office of the Chief Component Procurement Officer's cited efforts.

Therefore, we encourage FEMA's Head of Contracting Activity to take additional action to address the recommendation. Doing so will ensure that contracting lessons learned from COVID-19 and future emergencies are effectively captured and available to be shared as part of more formal lessons learned processes conducted by the Continuous Improvement Program.

In its response, OMB agreed with our fourth recommendation to update the Emergency Acquisitions Guide to account for information on the obstacles contracting officers may face when assessing prospective vendors during an emergency and key practices or resources to address those obstacles. OMB did not agree with our fifth recommendation, that OFPP establish a process and time frames for regularly updating the Emergency Acquisitions Guide to ensure resources and practices that can be used during an emergency are current. OMB stated that after it revises the guide in response to, among other things, our fourth recommendation, it plans to confer with other federal agencies about the best way to collect and share information. OMB said it does not want to assume that maintaining information in the current format of the Emergency Acquisitions Guide is the most effective form of communication. We continue to believe that establishing a process and time frames for updating the resources and practices available in the Emergency Acquisitions Guide—a tool agencies can use when contracting during emergencies—will ensure that federal agencies (particularly those not typically involved in emergency response activities) have the most up to date information to assist them. As noted in our findings, the guide and the resources it contains have not been updated since 2011, precluding agencies from the benefit of the experiences and practices other federal agencies have encountered in the numerous disasters and emergencies since then.

We are sending copies of this report to the appropriate congressional committees and offices; and the Secretaries of Defense, Health and Human Services, Agriculture, Veterans Affairs, and Homeland Security, and the Acting Director of OMB. In addition, the report will be made available at no charge on the GAO website at http://www.gao.gov.

If you or your staff have any questions concerning this report, please contact me at (202) 512-4841. Contact points for our offices of Congressional Relations and Public Affairs may be found on the last page of this report. Staff members making key contributions to this report are listed in appendix V.

Marie A. Mak
Director, Contracting and National Security Acquisitions

List of Addressees

The Honorable Patrick Leahy
Chairman

The Honorable Richard Shelby
Vice Chairman
Committee on Appropriations
United States Senate

The Honorable Ron Wyden
Chairman

The Honorable Mike Crapo
Ranking Member
Committee on Finance
United States Senate

The Honorable Patty Murray
Chair

The Honorable Richard Burr
Ranking Member
Committee on Health, Education, Labor, and Pensions
United States Senate

The Honorable Gary C. Peters
Chairman

The Honorable Rob Portman
Ranking Member
Committee on Homeland Security and Governmental Affairs
United States Senate

The Honorable Rosa L. DeLauro
Chairwoman

The Honorable Kay Granger
Ranking Member
Committee on Appropriations
House of Representatives

The Honorable Frank Pallone, Jr.
Chairman

The Honorable Cathy McMorris Rodgers
Republican Leader
Committee on Energy and Commerce
House of Representatives

The Honorable Bennie G. Thompson
Chair

The Honorable John Katko
Ranking Member
Committee on Homeland Security
House of Representatives

The Honorable Carolyn B. Maloney
Chairwoman

The Honorable James Comer
Ranking Member
Committee on Oversight and Reform
House of Representatives

The Honorable Richard E. Neal
Chair
The Honorable Kevin Brady
Republican Leader
Committee on Ways and Means
House of Representatives

The Honorable Chris Pappas
Chairman
Subcommittee on Oversight and Investigations Committee on Veterans' Affairs
House of Representatives

Appendix I: Objectives, Scope, and Methodology

The CARES Act included a provision for GAO to provide a comprehensive audit and review of federal contracting pursuant to authorities provided in the act.[1] This report examines (1) contract obligations and characteristics of vendors; (2) the information selected agencies used to assess prospective vendors and the extent to which the agencies communicated available information to contracting officers; and (3) the extent to which selected agencies experienced challenges and established processes to collect and share contracting lessons learned.

To identify contract obligations and the characteristics of vendors, we analyzed data available in the Federal Procurement Data System (FPDS) as of

[1] Pub. L. No. 116-136, div. B, tit. IX, § 19010, 134 Stat. 281, 579 (2020). We regularly issue government-wide reports on the federal response to COVID-19. For the latest report, see GAO, *COVID-19: Continued Attention Needed to Improve Federal Preparedness, Response, and Service Delivery and Enhance Program Integrity,* GAO-21-551 (Washington, D.C.: July 19, 2021). Our next government-wide report will be issued in October 2021 and will be available on GAO's website at https://www.gao.gov/coronavirus.

May 31, 2021.[2] Though agencies may obligate dollars through various other vehicles, such as grants or cooperative agreements, this report is focused specifically on contract obligations.[3] We primarily identified these contract actions and associated obligations related to the Coronavirus Disease 2019 (COVID-19) response by using the National Interest Action code.[4] We supplemented the use of the National Interest Action code by searching for "coronavirus" and "COVID-19" in the contract description field to identify a limited number of additional contractactions and associated obligations.[5] Some contract actions identified as being related to COVID-19 based on the National Interest Action code included obligations not specific to the pandemic.[6] Therefore, for contract actions over $1 million, we removed obligations that were identified in the contract description as not related to COVID-19. We assessed the reliability of FPDS data by reviewing existing information about the FPDS system and the data it collects—specifically, the data dictionary and data validation rules—and performing electronic testing. We determined the FPDS data were sufficiently reliable for the purposes of describing agencies' reported contract obligations to vendors in response to COVID- 19.

We analyzed the FPDS data to identify the agencies with the highest COVID-19 contract obligations, the types of goods and services procured, and

[2] We accessed FPDS data available on SAM.gov as of May 31, 2021. SAM.gov is the new System for Award Management and can perform functions of other federal government systems including FPDS.

[3] For the purposes of this report, "contract obligations" means obligations on contracts that are subject to the Federal Acquisition Regulation, and does not include, for example, grants, cooperative agreements, loans, other transactions for research, real property leases, or requisitions from federal stock.

[4] National Interest Action codes were established in 2005 after Hurricane Katrina with the purpose of tracking federal procurements for specific disasters, emergencies, or contingency events. A National Interest Action code was established on March 13, 2020 for the COVID-19 pandemic, and contract actions and their associated obligations are coded as related to the COVID-19 response in a field in FPDS.

[5] In November 2019, we identified some inconsistencies in the information agencies report in the contract description field in FPDS. See GAO, *DATA Act: Quality of Data Submissions Has Improved but Further Action Is Needed to Disclose Known Data Limitations*, GAO-20-75 (Washington, D.C.: Nov. 8, 2019). Data on DOD contract obligations based on information in the description field were available only through March 1, 2021, due to differences in the time frames for which DOD data are made publicly available.

[6] According to the Office of Management and Budget, any contract action affected by COVID-19 is to be reported using the National Interest Action code, including modifications that were issued to address COVID-19, irrespective of whether the contract being modified was originally awarded to address COVID-19. See Office of Management and Budget, M-20-21 *Implementation Guidance for Supplemental Funding Provided in Response to the Coronavirus Disease 2019 (COVID-19)* (Apr. 10, 2020).

other vendor characteristics such as whether a vendor had prior federal contracting experience—defined in terms of whether a vendor had any contract awards in the last 15 years—and whether the vendor was a small or large business. We also reviewed descriptions of contract modifications to identify cancelled obligations, or deobligations, such as for contract terminations. We used data from FPDS from calendar years 2005 through 2019 to evaluate the frequency agencies have historically awarded contracts to first time federal contractors in calendar years 2016 through 2020, compared to the contracts awarded in response to COVID-19. We augmented data from FPDS with data from the System for Award Management (SAM) to identify additional information about vendors receiving COVID-19 contracts, including whether or not vendors were registered in SAM. We also used data from the Federal Awardee Performance and Integrity Information System (FAPIIS) to identify vendors that had a performance or integrity information record in FAPIIS for prior performance or integrity concerns. We assessed the reliability ofSAM data by reviewing existing information about the data contained in the system—specifically, the SAM user guide—and performing electronic testing. We also assessed the reliability of FAPIIS data by performing electronic testing. We determined that both SAM and FAPIIS data were sufficiently reliable for the purposes of describing vendor registration status and prior records of unsatisfactory performance.

To determine what information selected agencies used to assess prospective vendors awarded contracts in response to COVID-19, we identified four of the top five departments with the highest COVID-19 contract obligations as of August 31, 2020—the Departments of Defense (DOD), Health and Human Services (HHS), Agriculture (USDA), and Homeland Security (DHS).[7] Within these departments, we selected the agencies that collectively accounted for at least two-thirds of each department's COVID-19 contract obligations:

- DOD's Defense Logistics Agency (DLA) and the Department of the Army;

[7] We selected August 31, 2020 as it was the time we were beginning and scoping our review. The other agency with the highest contract obligations was the Department of Veterans Affairs, which we did not include due to other ongoing work on the department's contracting response to COVID-19. See GAO, *VA COVID-19 Procurements: Pandemic Underscores Urgent Need to Modernize Supply Chain,* GAO-21-280 (Washington, D.C.: June 15, 2021).

- HHS's Office of the Assistant Secretary for Preparedness and Response (ASPR);
- USDA's Agricultural Marketing Service (AMS); and
- DHS's Federal Emergency Management Agency (FEMA).

We initially selected a nongeneralizable sample of eight COVID-19-related contracts and task or delivery orders with obligations or deobligations over $5 million (hereafter referred to as contracts, unless otherwise specified) per department, for a total of 32 contracts awarded between January 2020 and August 31, 2020. To obtain a mix of vendor and contract characteristics, we judgmentally selected five contracts from each department based on factors such as obligation or deobligation amount, whether the vendor had prior federal contracting experience, whether the vendor was registered in SAM.gov when the contract was awarded, whether the contract was competed, and the vendor's business size. After making those selections, we selected three other contracts from each department randomly. Subsequent to these selections, we removed four contracts from our review: three because they were potentially the subject of an ongoing Office of Inspector General or other federal investigation; and one because it was reported as awarded in FPDS, but agency officials told us it was never awarded. This left us with a total of 28 contracts—seven from each department.[8] See table 4 for additional details on the selected contracts included in our review.

To review our selected contracts, we gathered and reviewed contract documentation related to assessments of prospective vendors, such as vendor proposals, responsibility determinations (where available), and source selection evaluation reports. We also conducted semi-structured interviews with contracting officials responsible for the 28 selectedcontracts to discuss the resources they used to assess prospective vendors.

To assess the extent to which selected agencies communicated the information available to contracting officers to assess prospective vendors, we reviewed agency, department, and government-wide guidance and regulations related to assessing prospective vendors and emergency acquisitions. This included the Federal Acquisition Regulation (FAR), department and agency supplements to the FAR, agency guidance and job aids, and the Office of Management and Budget's Office of Federal Procurement Policy's (OFPP)

[8] For DOD, we selected three contracts from DLA and four from the Department of the Army. Within the Department of the Army, we selected one contract from Army Contracting Command and three contracts from the U.S. Army Corps of Engineers.

Emergency Acquisitions Guide. We also reviewed federal internal control standards on risk assessment, information, and communication.[9] We interviewed acquisition policy and contracting officials responsible for our selected contracts to determine contracting officers' awareness of information and resources available to assess prospective vendors during an emergency. We also interviewed OFPP staff to identify efforts, if any, underway to update or revise the Emergency Acquisitions Guide.

Table 4. Description of selected contracts

Awarding Agency	Description	Obligation Amount as of August 31, 2020	Vendor had prior federal contracting experience
Department of Defense			
Defense Logistics Agency	Services for operations, maintenance, and repairs of N95 respirator decontamination system	$147,595,011	X
Defense Logistics Agency	Personal protective equipment	$862,751,155	X
Defense Logistics Agency	Cloth face coverings	$5,372,000	X
Army Contracting Command	Reservation of vaccine fill and finish capacity	$160,000,000	-
U.S. Army Corps of Engineers	Construction of alternate care facilities	$8,300,000	X
U.S. Army Corps of Engineers	Construction of alternate care facilities	$700,000[a]	X
U.S. Army Corps of Engineers	Construction of alternate care facilities	$13,331,415	X
Department of Health and Human Services			
Assistant Secretary for Preparedness and Response	Ventilators	$646,683,750[b]	X
Assistant Secretary for Preparedness and Response	Surgical face masks	$0[a]	-
Assistant Secretary for Preparedness and Response	Cloth face masks	$55,250,000	-
Assistant Secretary for Preparedness and Response	N95 respirators	$31,241,700	X
Assistant Secretary for Preparedness and Response	Ventilators	$31,982,100	X
Assistant Secretary for Preparedness and Response	Reservation and expansion of vaccine manufacturing capacity	$264,693,063	X

[9] GAO, *Standards for Internal Control in the Federal Government*, GAO-14-704G (Washington, D.C.: September 2014).

Table 4. Continued

Awarding Agency	**Description**	**Obligation Amount as of August 31, 2020**	**Vendor had prior federal contracting experience**
Assistant Secretary for Preparedness and Response	Expansion of COVID-19 test production	$13,000,000	X
U.S. Department of Agriculture			
Agricultural Marketing Service	Fluid milk	$72,898,396	X
Agricultural Marketing Service	Fresh fruit and vegetable box	$12,220,000	-
Agricultural Marketing Service	Dairy products box, fluid milk	$16,596,997	-
Agricultural Marketing Service	Combination food box	$147,456,691	X
Agricultural Marketing Service	Fresh fruit and vegetable box	$40,000,000c	-
Agricultural Marketing Service	Fresh fruit and vegetable box	$6,916,536	-
Agricultural Marketing Service	Pre-cooked meat box	$22,001,720	-
Department of Homeland Security			
Federal Emergency Management Agency	Reusable knit and woven gowns	$543,155,000	-
Federal Emergency Management Agency	Powered air purifying respirators	$96,434,000	X
Federal Emergency Management Agency	N95 and KN95 respirators and disposable masks	$48,799,999	-
Federal Emergency Management Agency	N95 respirators	$0[a]	X
Federal Emergency Management Agency	Nitrile gloves and surgical masks	$5,860,000	X
Federal Emergency Management Agency	National medical transport and support services	$256,005,094	X
Federal Emergency Management Agency	Isolation gowns	$17,243,600	X

Source: GAO analysis of selected contract files and Federal Procurement Data System data. | GAO-21-528.

Legend:

X = vendor identified as having prior federal contracting experience.

- = vendor identified as not having prior federal contracting experience.

[a] Prior to August 31, 2020, the agency deobligated most or all of the funds for this contract. For each of these applicable contracts, the deobligations exceeded $5 million.

[b] The contract was partially terminated. A determination on the type of termination is pending.

[c] The contract was terminated for the government's convenience, and, according to agency officials, negotiations on the termination settlement are ongoing. Accordingly, the final obligation amount is pending.

To determine the extent to which selected agencies experienced challenges when contracting in response to COVID-19 and established processes to collect and share contracting lessons learned, we interviewed DOD, HHS, USDA, and DHS contracting officials for our 28 selected contracts to identify the challenges they faced, if any, during the response to COVID-19. We reviewed available COVID-19 after-action reports at DOD, USDA, and DHS to identify agencies' lessons learned and proposed actions to address these lessons.[10] We also interviewed contracting officials at each agency or department and officials responsible for gathering and reporting on lessons learned to assess their efforts to collect and share lessons against leading practices we and others have previously identified.[11]

We conducted this performance audit from August 2020 to July 2021 in accordance with generally accepted government auditing standards.

Those standards require that we plan and perform the audit to obtain sufficient, appropriate evidence to provide a reasonable basis for our findings and conclusions based on our audit objectives. We believe that the evidence obtained provides a reasonable basis for our findings and conclusions based on our audit objectives.

---

[10] HHS had not completed an after-action report at the time of our review.

[11] GAO, Army Modernization: Army Should Improve Use of Alternative Agreements and Approaches by Enhancing Oversight and Communication of Lessons Learned, GAO-21-8 (Washington, D.C.: Oct. 1, 2020); DOD Utilities Privatization: Improved Data Collection and Lessons Learned Archive Could Help Reduce Time to Award Contracts, GAO-20-104 (Washington, D.C.; Apr. 2, 2020); Project Management: DOE and NNSA Should Improve Their Lessons-Learned Process for Capital Asset Projects, GAO-19-25 (Washington, D.C.: Dec. 21, 2018); and Federal Real Property Security: Interagency Security Committee Should Implement a Lessons-Learned Process, GAO-12-901 (Washington, D.C.: Sept. 10, 2012). GAO-19-25 identified some lessons learned practices from reports by both the Project Management Institute and Department of the Army, Combined Arms Center, Center for Army Lessons Learned. Project Management Institute, Inc., A Guide to the Project Management Body of Knowledge (PMBOK® Guide), Sixth Edition, 2017; Project Management Institute, Inc., Implementing Organizational Project Management: A Practice Guide, First Edition, 2014; and Center for Army Lessons Learned, Establishing a Lessons Learned Program: Observations, Insights, and Lessons (Fort Leavenworth, KS: June 2011).

Appendix II: Comments from the Department of Defense

OFFICE OF THE UNDER SECRETARY OF DEFENSE
3000 DEFENSE PENTAGON
WASHINGTON, DC 20301-3000

ACQUISITION
AND SUSTAINMENT

JUL 13 2021

Ms. Marie Mak
Director, Contracting and National Security
U.S. Government Accountability Office
441 G Street, NW
Washington DC 20548

Dear Ms. Mak,

This is the Department of Defense response to GAO-21-528 Draft Report, "COVID-19 CONTRACTING: Opportunities to Improve Practices to Assess Prospective Vendors and Capture Lessons Learned," dated June 22, 2021 (GAO Code 104499).

Enclosed is the Department's response to the subject report. My point of contact is Mr. Gregory Snyder who can be reached at gregory.d.snyder.civ@mail.mil or 703-614-0719.

Sincerely,

for John M. Tenaglia
Principal Director,
Defense Pricing and Contracting

Enclosure:
As stated

Eclosure

GAO DRAFT REPORT DATED JUNE 22, 2021
GAO-21-528 (GAO CODE 104499)

"COVID-19 CONTRACTING: OPPORTUNITIES TO IMPROVE PRACTICES TO ASSESS PROSPECTIVE VENDORS AND CAPTURE LESSONS LEARNED"

DEPARTMENT OF DEFENSE COMMENTS
TO THE GAO RECOMMENDATION

RECOMMENDATION 8: The Secretary of Defense, in coordination with the Secretaries of Homeland Security and Health and Human Services, should ensure that input from contracting officials on interagency contracting lessons learned in response to COVID-19 is collected and shared as part of government-wide efforts to collect, analyze, and report on lessons learned.

DoD RESPONSE: Concur. The Department will collect, analyze, and report it's interagency contracting lessons learned and share those with the Departments of Homeland Security (DHS) and Health and Human Services (HHS).

Appendix III: Comments from the Department of Health and Human Services

DEPARTMENT OF HEALTH & HUMAN SERVICES

OFFICE OF THE SECRETARY

Assistant Secretary for Legislation
Washington, DC 20201

July 15, 2021

Marie Mak
Director, Contracting and National Security Acquisitions
U.S. Government Accountability Office
441 G Street NW
Washington, DC 20548

Dear Ms. Mak:

Attached are comments on the U.S. Government Accountability Office's (GAO) report entitled, *"Opportunities to Improve Practices to Assess Prospective Vendors and Capture Lessons Learned"* (Job code 104499/GAO-21-528).

The Department appreciates the opportunity to review this report prior to publication.

Sincerely,

Jeff Hild
Acting Assistant Secretary for Legislation
Principal Deputy Assistant Secretary for Legislation

Attachment

GENERAL COMMENTS FROM THE DEPARTMENT OF HEALTH & HUMAN SERVICES ON THE GOVERNMENT ACCOUNTABILITY OFFICE'S DRAFT REPORT ENTITLED OPPORTUNITIES TO IMPROVE PRACTICES TO ASSESS PROSPECTIVE VENDORS AND CAPTURE LESSONS LEARNED (GAO-21-528)

The U.S. Department of Health & Human Services (HHS) appreciates the opportunity from the Government Accountability Office (GAO) to review and comment on this draft report.

Recommendation 1
The Secretary of Health and Human Services should direct the Assistant Secretary for Preparedness and Response to review and fully communicate the resources available to contracting officers for assessing prospective vendors—including resources to assess financial capability. **(Recommendation 1)**

HHS Response
HHS concurs with GAO's recommendation.

In making the determination of responsibility, SNS Contracting Officers (CO) did comply with **FAR Subpart 9.0 Contractor Qualifications and HHS Acquisition Regulation 309.404** when considering information available to determine contractor's qualification or responsibility.

FAPIIS and CPARS are linked to beta.sam.gov. Therefore, pulling the beta.sam report provided the CO with performance data contained in FAPIIS and CPARS. Additionally, SNS COs complied with FAR Subpart 9.104.5. Representations and Certifications regarding responsibility matters were properly included in the commercial contracts IAW 52.209-5-Certification Regarding Responsibility Matters or paragraph (h) of provision 52.212-3. This clause references criteria in determining financial integrity and performance criteria for contractors.

Recommendation 2
The Secretary of Health and Human Services should direct the Assistant Secretary for Preparedness and Response to develop internal guidance that includes information for contracting officers related to contracting and assessing prospective vendors during emergencies. **(Recommendation 2)**

HHS Response
HHS concurs with GAO's recommendation.

ASPR Contracting Officers follow the FAR for all parts of the contracting process.

Recommendation 6
The Secretary of Health and Human Services should ensure that, as part of the Exercise, Evaluation and After Actions Division's ongoing after-action reporting and corrective action program, contracting lessons learned in response to COVID-19 and future emergency response efforts are collected, analyzed, validated, archived, and shared to inform HHS's contracting efforts in response to ongoing and future emergencies. **(Recommendation 6)**

Page **1** of **2**

GENERAL COMMENTS FROM THE DEPARTMENT OF HEALTH & HUMAN SERVICES ON THE GOVERNMENT ACCOUNTABILITY OFFICE'S DRAFT REPORT ENTITLED OPPORTUNITIES TO IMPROVE PRACTICES TO ASSESS PROSPECTIVE VENDORS AND CAPTURE LESSONS LEARNED (GAO-21-528)

HHS Response
HHS concurs with GAO's recommendation.

HHS will continue to utilize the Exercise, Evaluation and After Actions Division's after-action reporting and corrective action program to collect, analyze, validate, archive, and share information from HHS's contracting efforts in response to ongoing and future emergencies.

Recommendation 9
The Secretary of Health and Human Services, in coordination with the Secretaries of Defense and Homeland Security, should ensure that input from contracting officials on interagency contracting lessons learned in response to COVID-19 is collected and shared as part of government-wide efforts to collect, analyze, and report on lessons learned. **(Recommendation 9)**

HHS Response
HHS concurs with GAO's recommendation.

The HHS Exercise, Evaluation and After Actions Division will collect, within DHHS, any interagency contracting lessons learned and share those with the Departments of Defense (DoD) and Department of Homeland Security (DHS). HHS will work with DoD and HHS to develop a consolidated list of lessons learned and share those with any government-wide efforts to report on lessons learned.

Appendix IV: Comments from the Department of Homeland Security

U.S. Department of Homeland Security
Washington, DC 20528

Homeland Security

July 14, 2021

Marie A. Mak
Director, Contracting and National Security Acquisitions
U.S. Government Accountability Office
441 G Street, NW
Washington, DC 20548

Re: Management Response to Draft Report GAO-21-528, "COVID-19 CONTRACTING: Opportunities to Improve Practices to Assess Prospective Vendors and Capture Lessons Learned"

Dear Ms. Mak:

Thank you for the opportunity to comment on this draft report. The U.S. Department of Homeland Security (DHS or the Department) appreciates the U.S. Government Accountability Office's (GAO) work in planning and conducting its review and issuing this report.

The Department is pleased to note GAO's recognition of several resources DHS developed to assist contracting officers in assessing prospective vendors. Specifically, the report highlights DHS's issuance of the DHS Responsibility Determination Job Aid, which is a tool for contracting professionals use to better assess the present responsibility of unknown vendors or those presenting increased risk to successful contract performance. The job aid provides contracting professionals with additional areas to consider in such circumstances, as well as identifying types of evidence that may be requested and analyzed to either confirm or mitigate identified concerns. DHS remains committed to effectively communicating resources and guidance for assessing prospective vendors and collecting and sharing contracting lessons learned that could help inform future emergency response efforts.

The draft report contained ten recommendations, including two for DHS with which the Department concurs. Attached find our detailed response to each recommendation. DHS previously submitted technical comments addressing several accuracy, contextual, and other issues under a separate cover for GAO's consideration.

Again, thank you for the opportunity to review and comment on this draft report. Please feel free to contact me if you have any questions. We look forward to working with you again in the future.

Sincerely,

JIM H CRUMPACKER Digitally signed by JIM H CRUMPACKER
Date: 2021.07.14 09:41:01 -04'00'

JIM H. CRUMPACKER, CIA, CFE
Director
Departmental GAO-OIG Liaison Office

Attachment

Attachment: Management Response to Recommendations Contained in GAO-21-528

GAO recommended that the Administrator of the Federal Emergency Management Agency (FEMA):

Recommendation 7: Direct the Head of [the] Contracting Activity [HCA] to establish a formal process to (1) collect contracting lessons learned from COVID-19 and future emergency response efforts; and (2) ensure contracting lessons learned are shared with the Continuous Improvement Program [CIP] for inclusion in FEMA's formal lessons learned process to inform FEMA's contracting efforts in response to ongoing and future emergencies.

Response: Concur. FEMA's CIP, located in the National Preparedness Directorate, conducted extensive interviews, analysis, and notetaking regarding lessons learned from COVID-19, including interviews of the FEMA HCA and Deputy Head of the Contracting Activity. These findings were published in the "Pandemic Response to Coronavirus Disease 2019 (COVID-19): Initial Assessment Report for FEMA Operations January Through September 2020," dated January 2021. It is important to note that not all interviews conducted as part of the CIP process necessarily lead to an official observation or finding in final agency reports, but the work is nevertheless conducted as part of the data collection process and results are available to leadership, program officials, subject matter experts, and others for their information and use as deemed appropriate.

FEMA's CIP also provides evaluation, advisory and decision support, and process improvement services to each of FEMA's program areas to help facilitate effectiveness and efficiency improvements where possible. For example, the CIP serves as the official and authoritative entity within FEMA to capture lessons learned for inclusion into formal agency after action reports, such as the aforementioned COVID-19 Initial Assessment Report, the "2017 Hurricane Season FEMA After-Action Report," dated July 12, 2018, and other reports that are used to help inform ongoing and future emergency response efforts.

Additionally, FEMA's Office of the Chief Component Procurement Officer: (1) conducts internal hot washes; (2) holds Contracting Officer Representative (COR) Engagement Sessions on a quarterly basis to disseminate information; (3) conducts open dialogue surrounding COR challenging situations; and (4) captures internal lessons learned following major disaster operations to continually refine contracting processes and procedures as applicable.

Given these established roles, relationships, and processes, FEMA believes standardized mechanisms currently exist that sufficiently collect and share lessons learned. DHS requests that GAO consider this recommendation resolved and closed, as implemented.

GAO recommended that the Secretary of Homeland Security, in coordination with the Secretaries of Defense and Health and Human Services [HHS]:

Recommendation 10: Ensure that input from contracting officials on interagency contracting lessons learned in response to COVID-19 is collected and shared as part of government-wide efforts to collect, analyze, and report on lessons learned.

Response: Concur. The DHS Office of the Chief Procurement Officer (OCPO) will collect, within DHS, any interagency contracting lessons learned and share those with the Department of Defense (DoD) and HHS. As part of this effort, OCPO will work with DoD and HHS to develop a consolidated list of lessons learned and share those as part of any government-wide effort(s) to report on lessons learned. ECD: March 31, 2022.

4

Appendix V: Staff Acknowledgments

In addition to the contact named above, Janet McKelvey (Assistant Director), Meghan Perez (Analyst in Charge), Dennis Antonio, Matthew T. Crosby, Lorraine Ettaro, Betsy Gregory-Hosler, Stephanie Gustafson, Julia Kennon, Sarah Tempel, and Robin Wilson made key contributions to this report.

Chapter 2

COVID-19 Contracting: Actions Needed to Enhance Transparency and Oversight of Selected Awards*

United States Government Accountability Office

Why GAO Did This Study

In March 2020, Congress passed the CARES Act as part of the federal response to COVID-19. The act had certain provisions for federal contracting, including providing additional flexibilities. Contracting plays a critical role in the pandemic response as agencies obligate billions of dollars for goods and services.

The act also included a provision for GAO to review federal contracting in response to COVID-19. This report examines, among other objectives, the extent to which the Departments of Defense, Health and Human Services, and Homeland Security—the only agencies that reported using other transaction agreements in response to COVID-19 in the federal procurement database—used such agreements, including awards to consortia, and oversight of such use.

GAO analyzed federal procurement data as of March 2021; reviewed a nongeneralizable sample of 15 agreements selected based on high dollar amounts, agency, a mix of products and services, among other criteria; reviewed agency policies; and interviewed agency officials.

---

* This is an edited, reformatted and augmented version of Report to Congressional Committees, Publication No. GAO-21-501, dated July 2021.

In: COVID-19 Contracting
Editor: Eric Neudorf
ISBN: 978-1-68507-710-5

What GAO Recommends

GAO is making 14 recommendations to selected agencies, to improve the transparency of agreement awards in the federal procurement database and update policies to improve the oversight of agreements awarded through consortium management firms. The agencies agreed with 11 of the recommendations and did not agree with three of them. GAO continues to believe the recommendations are valid, as discussed in the report.

What GAO Found

In response to COVID-19, as of March 2021, the Departments of Defense, Health and Human Services, and Homeland Security obligated at least $12.5 billion using a contracting mechanism that gave them the flexibility to quickly respond to urgent pandemic needs. This mechanism—known as an other transaction agreement—is not subject to certain federal contract laws and requirements but allowed the agencies to customize the agreements. Agencies cited the timeliness of awards as a major factor for using these agreements, including awards that accelerated COVID-19 vaccine manufacturing.

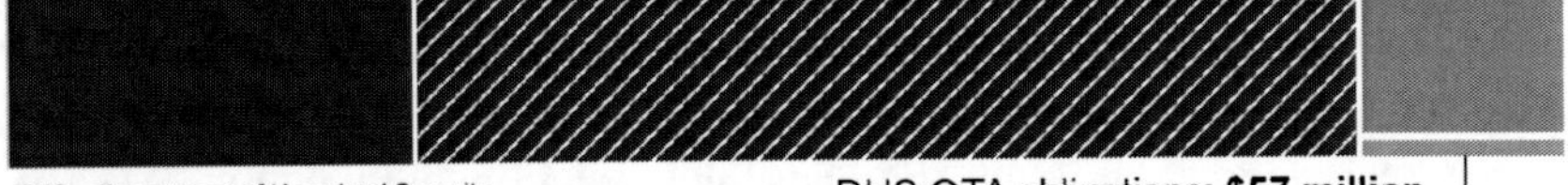
Total COVID-19 OTA Obligations are $12.5 billion
DOD OTA obligations
$10.9 billion
OTA consortium obligations
$7.2 billion
HHS OTA
obligations
$1.6 billion
DHS OTA obligations: $57 million

DHS = Department of Homeland Security
DOD = Department of Defense
FPDS-NG = Federal Procurement Data System-Next Generation
HHS = Department of Health and Human Services
OTA = Other transaction agreement

Source: GAO analysis of FPDS-NG data and information from DOD, HHS, and DHS. | GAO-21-501.

Obligations on Other Transaction Agreements in Response to COVID-19 as of March 2021.

The Department of Defense used this mechanism to award $7.2 billion to consortium members—organizations and federal contractors organized around a specific topic area—through one consortium management firm (see figure).

GAO's analysis found two challenges with how the agencies tracked these agreements due to limitations with the federal procurement database. First, the three agencies did not properly identify at least $1.6 billion of the $12.5 billion as COVID-19-related agreements. Second, the Department of Defense reported that one consortium management firm received $7.2 billion in agreements, as noted above. In actuality, the management firm distributed nearly all of the awarded dollars to five pharmaceutical companies, with each receiving $450 million to $2 billion. The database is the only way for Congress and the public to track these obligations, but transparency is limited without accurate reporting.

Also, two agencies' policies on other transaction agreements did not address the requirement for enhanced oversight of certain activities that consortium management firms may perform, potentially posing risks to the government. According to Office of Federal Procurement Policy guidance, these types of activities require enhanced oversight because they can closely support tasks fundamental to the public interest, such as the award of contracts. By not addressing such oversight in their policies, agencies may not fully consider the range of actions they should take to mitigate risks of inappropriate influence for government decisions.

Abbreviations

ASPR	Office of the Assistant Secretary for Preparedness and Response
ATI	Advanced Technology International
COVID-19	Coronavirus Disease 2019
DHS	Department of Homeland Security
DOD	Department of Defense
GSA	General Services Administration
FAR	Federal Acquisition Regulation
FPDS-NG	Federal Procurement Data System-Next Generation
HHS	Department of Health and Human Services
OTA	other transaction agreement

July 26, 2021
Congressional Committees

The Coronavirus Disease 2019 (COVID-19) pandemic has resulted in catastrophic loss of life and substantial damage to the global economy. In the U.S., there have been over 33 million reported cases and over 595,000 reported deaths due to COVID-19 as of July 2, 2021.[1] The country also continues to experience serious economic repercussions. Among other actions in response to this unprecedented global crisis, in March 2020, Congress passed, and the President signed into law, the CARES Act, which provided over $2 trillion in emergency assistance and health care response for individuals, families, and businesses affected by COVID-19. The CARES Act also provided supplemental appropriations for federal agencies to respond to COVID-19 and included a number of provisions related to federal contracting efforts to facilitate agencies' responses to the pandemic. Federal contracting continues to play a critical role in the response to COVID-19. Agencies have obligated nearly $69 billion as of March 2021 through a variety of contracting mechanisms to acquire vital goods and services.

One type of contracting mechanism, called other transaction agreements (OTA), has played a significant role in the response to COVID-19. Unlike procurement contracts, OTAs are not subject to federal acquisition regulations. The CARES Act removed certain requirements related to the use of OTAs for the Department of Health and Human Services (HHS) and the Department of Defense (DOD), such as requirements related to congressional reporting and who can approve certain OTAs.[2] The CARES Act also relaxed certain limitations on DOD's use of undefinitized contracts—a procurement contract mechanism that is subject to federal and DOD acquisition regulations and allows contractors to begin work before all terms and conditions are finalized.[3]

---

[1] Data on COVID-19 cases are based on aggregate case reporting to the Centers for Disease Control and Prevention and include probable and confirmed cases as reported by states and jurisdictions. The Centers for Disease Control and Prevention's National Center for Health Statistics COVID-19 death counts in the U.S. are based on provisional counts from death certificate data, which do not distinguish between laboratory-confirmed and probable COVID-19 deaths.

[2] Pub. L. No. 116-136, §§ 3301, 13006, 134 Stat. at 383, 522.

[3] Pub. L. No. 116-136, § 13005, 134 Stat. at 522. See also Defense Federal Acquisition Regulation Supplement subpt. 217.74.

The CARES Act includes a provision for GAO to conduct a comprehensive audit and review of federal contracting pursuant to authorities provided in the act.[4] This report is one in a series of reports in response to that provision.[5] This report examines the extent to which: (1) selected agencies used OTAs in response to COVID-19 and what factors contributed to their use, (2) these COVID-19 OTAs were awarded to consortia and how agencies provided oversight, and (3) selected agencies used and managed undefinitized contracts in response to COVID-19.

To identify the extent to which selected agencies used OTAs in response to COVID-19, we identified all the agencies that reported obligating dollars through OTAs in response to COVID-19 in the Federal Procurement Database System-Next Generation (FPDS-NG), as of March 14, 2021.[6] These agencies were:

- DOD;[7]

---

[4] Pub. L. No. 116-136, § 19010. The CARES Act also requires GAO to, among other things, conduct monitoring and oversight of the exercise of authorities, or the receipt, disbursement, and use of funds made available by law to prepare for, respond to, and recover from the pandemic. We regularly issue government-wide reports on the federal response to COVID-19. For the latest report, see GAO, *COVID-19: Continued Attention Needed to Enhance Federal Preparedness, Response, Service Delivery, and Program Integrity,* GAO-21-551 (Washington, D.C.: July 19, 2021). Our next government-wide report will be issued in October 2021 and will be available on GAO's website at https://www.gao.gov/coronavirus.

[5] For COVID-19 contracting reports, see GAO, *VA COVID-19 Procurements: Pandemic Underscores Urgent Need to Modernize Supply Chain,* GAO-21-280 (Washington, D.C.: June 15, 2021); *COVID-19: Efforts to Increase Vaccine Availability and Perspectives on Initial Implementation,* GAO-21-443 (Washington, D.C.: Apr. 14, 2021); *Defense Production Act: Opportunities Exist to Increase Transparency and Identify Future Actions to Mitigate Medical Supply Chain Issues,* GAO-21-108 (Washington, D.C.: Nov. 19, 2020); *COVID-19 Contracting: Observations on Contractor Paid Leave Reimbursement Guidance and Use,* GAO-20-662 (Washington, D.C.: Sept. 3, 2020); and *COVID-19 Contracting: Observations on Federal Contracting in Response to the Pandemic*, GAO-20-632 (Washington, D.C.: July 29, 2020). We plan to issue future products focused on contractor paid leave reimbursement and agencies' assessment of prospective vendors and contracting lessons learned in response to the pandemic.

[6] FPDS-NG is a comprehensive, web-based tool for agencies to report procurement contract actions and is the authoritative source for procurement award data, including dollars obligated on contract actions. It also includes a module for reporting OTAs. In June 2021, FPDS-NG was renamed to FPDS. For the purposes of this report, we refer to the system as FPDS-NG.

[7] While DOD has authority to use OTAs for research, prototyping, and production purposes, this report is focused on OTAs used to support DOD's prototyping and production efforts.

- HHS—specifically, the Office of the Assistant Secretary for Preparedness and Response (ASPR), which includes the Biomedical Advanced Research and Development Authority;[8] and
- Department of Homeland Security (DHS)—specifically, the Countering Weapons of Mass Destruction Office and the Transportation Security Administration.

We analyzed the FPDS-NG data to identify the types of goods or services procured by DOD, HHS, and DHS using OTAs. We assessed the reliability of the FPDS-NG data by comparing them to OTA documentation and agency-provided data and by performing electronic testing, among other steps, and found the agencies did not accurately report all COVID-19 OTA obligations, which we discuss in the report. We identified additional COVID-19 OTA obligations through agency-provided data and documents. After we corrected the FPDS-NG OTA data for the inaccuracies and underreporting, we determined the data were sufficiently reliable for the purposes of describing agencies' reported OTA obligations in response to COVID-19. We also interviewed officials from the General Services Administration (GSA), which administers FPDS-NG, including the OTA module.

To identify the factors that contributed to DOD, HHS, and DHS using OTAs in selected cases, we selected a nongeneralizable sample of 15 OTAs awarded between February 2020 and October 2020. Our selections were based on the highest dollars obligated, representation of all three contracting agencies, and a mix of product or service acquired, among other criteria. When we selected our sample of OTAs in October 2020, the obligations on all COVID-19 OTAs across DOD, HHS, and DHS were 30 percent of total obligations for these three agencies. We selected all seven vaccine OTAs awarded by DOD and HHS, which comprised $8.9 billion in obligations. We also selected eight nonvaccine OTAs awarded by DOD, HHS, and DHS, which accounted for an additional $1.2 billion in obligations. Combined, these 15 OTAs accounted for 81 percent of all obligations on COVID-19 OTAs as of March 14, 2021. For these selected cases, we analyzed OTA documents, such as written determinations for OTA use, and interviewed agreements officers— federal employees with the authority to bind the government by

---

8 The National Institutes of Health—a part of HHS—did not report awarding any OTAs in response to COVID-19 in FPDS-NG as of March 14, 2021. In May 2021, officials from the National Institutes of Health informed us they had obligated about $520 million on COVID-19 OTAs as of April 26, 2021. We did not assess the reliability of these data and did not include the $520 million in our analysis.

signing an OTA—and program officials. As part of our analysis, we determined the extent to which these OTAs used available CARES Act flexibilities. In addition, we reviewed agencies' OTA policies and guidance and interviewed contracting policy officials at DOD, HHS, and DHS.

To identify the extent to which DOD, HHS, and DHS awarded OTAs to consortia in response to COVID-19, we analyzed the same data available in the OTA module of FPDS-NG discussed above by vendor. We supplemented this analysis with reviews of publicly available information and OTA documents. Of the 15 OTA cases we reviewed, six were awarded to consortia by DOD. To determine how DOD provided oversight for these six OTAs, we analyzed OTA documents and interviewed agreements officers and program officials. We reviewed DOD, HHS, and DHS policies related to OTAs awarded to consortia and these agencies' reports to congressional committees regarding OTA use. We also interviewed officials from Advanced Technology International (ATI), the consortium management firm that received the majority of COVID-19 OTA obligations according to FPDS-NG data.

To identify the extent to which DOD, HHS, and DHS used undefinitized contracts in response to COVID-19, we analyzed data available in the procurement contract module of FPDS-NG as of March 14, 2021. For the purposes of our data analysis, undefinitized contract obligations are associated with contract actions identified in FPDS-NG as undefinitized, which includes letter contracts. DOD, HHS, and DHS accounted for 96 percent of all COVID-19-related undefinitized contract obligations reported across the federal government over the time frame of our review.[9] We analyzed the FPDS-NG data to identify the types of goods or services procured by DOD, HHS, and DHS using undefinitized contracts. We assessed the reliability of the FPDS-NG data by comparing them to contract documentation and agency-provided data and performing electronic testing, among other steps, and determined that they were sufficiently reliable for the purposes of describing agencies' reported undefinitized obligations in response to COVID-19.

To identify how DOD, HHS, and DHS managed selected undefinitized contracts, we selected a nongeneralizable sample of three undefinitized contracts awarded between February 2020 and October 2020. Our selections were based on the highest dollars obligated, representation of the contracting

---

[9] On April 12, 2021, in response to our review, HHS corrected information for an undefinitized contract we reviewed by revising nine actions from being incorrectly identified as undefinitized to correctly identified as definitized. We updated our March 14, 2021 data analysis, which resulted in a reduction of HHS undefinitized contract obligations by $120 million.

agencies with the majority of undefinitized contract obligations (DOD and HHS), and a mix of product or service acquired, among other criteria. When we selected our sample of undefinitized contracts, the obligations on all COVID-19 undefinitized contracts across the three agencies were 6 percent of their total obligations during this time frame. The three undefinitized contracts we selected were awarded by DOD and HHS and had combined obligations of $509 million, or about 10 percent of all COVID-19 undefinitized contract obligations. For these selected cases, we analyzed contract documents, such as written determinations and award documents, and interviewed contracting officers and program officials. As part of our analysis, we determined the extent to which DOD used available CARES Act flexibilities for its undefinitized contracts. In addition, we reviewed federal acquisition regulations, agencies' federal acquisition regulation supplements, and agency policies and guidance related to undefinitized contracts. We also interviewed contracting policy officials at DOD, HHS, and DHS.

For additional information on our objectives, scope, and methodology, see appendix I.

We conducted this performance audit from August 2020 to July 2021 in accordance with generally accepted government auditing standards. Those standards require that we plan and perform the audit to obtain sufficient, appropriate evidence to provide a reasonable basis for our findings and conclusions based on our audit objectives. We believe that the evidence obtained provides a reasonable basis for our findings and conclusions based on our audit objectives.

Background

Every agency has inherent authority to award procurement contracts—contracts subject to the Federal Acquisition Regulation (FAR)—to procure goods or services for its own use. However, agencies must receive specific authority through legislation to award OTAs, which are not subject to the FAR. Undefinitized contracts are procurement contracts subject to the FAR but have certain requirements related to their use.

Overview of Other Transaction Agreements

OTAs are not required to include terms and conditions that are typically required when using procurement contracts subject to the FAR. They enable agencies and companies to start with a "blank sheet of paper" to negotiate contractual terms and conditions specific to the OTA. This flexibility can help agencies address concerns from nontraditional contractors—entities that do not typically do business with the federal government such as start-up companies—about requirements that apply to federal procurement contracts. These concerns can include establishing a government-unique cost accounting system or losing intellectual property rights, among others.[10] Our prior work found that OTAs with nontraditional companies have been used for research, prototyping, and production of new technologies or products.[11] We also found, however, risks with the use of OTAs regarding reduced accountability and transparency, in part, because they are exempt from the FAR and related oversight mechanisms that apply to procurement contracts.[12]

Congress provided the agencies in our review the authority to use OTAs, and each authority is unique to the agency:

- *DOD.* DOD generally has department-wide authority to award OTAs for research, prototyping, and production purposes. Specifically, DOD can use OTAs to carry out certain prototype projects, including those that are directly relevant to enhancing the mission effectiveness of military personnel and the supporting platforms, systems, components, or materials proposed to be acquired or developed by

---

[10] GAO, *Military Acquisitions: DOD Is Taking Steps to Address Challenges Faced by Certain Companies,* GAO-17-644 (Washington, D.C.: July 20, 2017).

[11] GAO, *Army Modernization: Army Should Improve Use of Alternative Agreements and Approaches by Enhancing Oversight and Communication of Lessons Learned,* GAO-21-8 (Washington, D.C.: Oct. 1, 2020); *Defense Acquisitions: DOD's Use of Other Transactions for Prototype Projects Has Increased,* GAO-20-84 (Washington, D.C.: Nov. 22, 2019); and *Federal Acquisitions: Use of 'Other Transaction' Agreements Limited and Mostly for Research and Development Activities,* GAO-16-209 (Washington, D.C.: Jan. 7, 2016).

[12] GAO, *COVID-19: Critical Vaccine Distribution, Supply Chain, Program Integrity, and Other Challenges Require Focused Federal Attention,* GAO-21-265 (Washington, D.C.: Jan. 28, 2021); *Transportation Security Administration: After Oversight Lapses, Compliance with Policy Governing Special Authority Has Been Strengthened,* GAO-18-172 (Washington, D.C.: Dec. 21, 2017); *Department of Homeland Security: Further Action Needed to Improve Management of Special Acquisition Authority,* GAO-12-557 (Washington, D.C.: May 8, 2012); and *Department of Homeland Security: Improvements Could Further Enhance Ability to Acquire Innovative Technologies Using Other Transaction Authority,* GAO-08-1088 (Washington, D.C.: Sept. 23, 2008).

DOD. DOD may not enter into a prototype OTA unless at least one of four conditions is met. The conditions are related to participation by a nontraditional defense contractor, nonprofit research institution or small business participation; cost sharing; or senior procurement executive approval.[13] Congress did not define a prototype project in statute, but DOD's November 2018 OTA guide defined a prototype project as addressing certain needs, such as a proof of concept, model, and novel application of commercial technologies for defense purposes. DOD can also award follow-on production OTAs—without using competitive procedures—to the participants of a competitively awarded prototype OTA, provided several conditions are met, such as successful completion of the prototype.[14]

Further, DOD agreements officers can award certain higher-dollar prototype OTAs if senior DOD contracting officials approve the OTAs in writing.[15] For example, for most DOD entities, OTAs expected to cost more than $100 million but not more than $500 million may only be carried out if the senior procurement executive makes a written determination that certain statutory requirements will be met and that use of OTA authority is essential to promoting the success of the prototype project.[16] OTAs expected to cost more than $500 million may only be carried out if the Under Secretary of Defense for Research and Engineering or the Under Secretary of Defense for Acquisition and Sustainment makes a written determination that certain statutory requirements will be met and that the use of OTA authority is essential to meet critical national security objectives. DOD must also notify the congressional defense committees in writing of any OTAs expected to cost more than $500 million at least 30 days before the OTA authority is exercised.

---

[13] National Defense Authorization Act for Fiscal Year 2016, Pub. L. No. 114-92, § 815 (2015), codified at 10 U.S.C. § 2371b. For purposes of DOD OTAs, a nontraditional defense contractor is an entity that is not performing on any DOD contract or subcontract that is subject to full coverage under the cost accounting standards prescribed by certain statutes and regulations, and has not performed on such a contract or subcontract for at least 1 year before DOD's solicitation for the OTA. 10 U.S.C. § 2302(9). The OTA authorities for HHS, the Transportation Security Administration, and DHS's Countering Weapons of Mass Destruction Office did not include statutory definitions of nontraditional contractors.

[14] 10 U.S.C. § 2371b(f).

[15] 10 U.S.C. § 2371b(a)(2).

[16] In the case of the Defense Advanced Research Projects Agency or the Missile Defense Agency, the agency director must make the written determination.

- *HHS.* Two of HHS's components have authority to award OTAs: ASPR, which leads the nation's response to public health emergencies and includes the Biomedical Advanced Research and Development Authority, and the National Institutes of Health, which is composed of 27 institutes and centers, each with a specific agenda.[17] ASPR's OTA authority supports advanced research and development for medical countermeasures, such as vaccines and therapeutics.[18] Several programs and types of projects within the National Institutes of Health have OTA authority, such as a program focused on researching heart, lung, and blood diseases.[19]
  ASPR's agreements officers can award OTAs expected to cost more than $100 million if the HHS Assistant Secretary for Financial Resources makes a written determination that use of such authority is essential to promoting the success of the project.[20]
- *DHS.* Two of DHS's components each have unique, unrestricted authorities to award OTAs to carry out their missions: the Countering Weapons of Mass Destruction Office and the Transportation Security Administration.[21] DHS also awards OTAs for research and prototyping efforts across the department.

The CARES Act removed certain requirements related to the use of OTAs for DOD and HHS ASPR in response to COVID-19, which we refer to as CARES Act flexibilities for the purposes of our report.[22] These flexibilities allow for delegation of OTA award approval to lower-level contracting officials and changes to congressional notification requirements.

Specifically, for DOD:

- Senior procurement executives can delegate approval of written determinations to other officials for prototype OTAs expected to cost more than $100 million but not more than $500 million.

---

[17] To fulfill its mission to seek fundamental knowledge about the nature and behavior of living systems and the application of that knowledge to enhance health, lengthen life, and reduce illness and disability, the National Institutes of Health funds research related to life processes and many diseases and conditions.

[18] 42 U.S.C. § 247d-7e(c)(5)(A).

[19] 42 U.S.C. § 285b-3; Consolidated and Further Continuing Appropriations Act, 2015, Pub. L No. 113-235, div. G, title II, § 213,128 Stat. 2487 (2014); 42 U.S.C. § 284n; and 42 U.S.C. § 287a.

[20] 42 U.S.C. § 247d-7e(c)(5)(A)(ii).

[21] 6 U.S.C. § 596 and 49 U.S.C. § 114(m).

[22] Pub. L. No. 116-136, §§ 3301, 13006, 134 Stat. at 383, 522.

- The Under Secretary of Defense for Research and Engineering and the Under Secretary of Defense for Acquisition and Sustainment can delegate approval of written determinations to other officials for prototype OTAs expected to cost more than $500 million.
- DOD can notify the congressional defense committees in writing of prototype OTAs expected to cost more than $500 million as soon as practicable after the OTA is awarded instead of at least 30 days before the OTA authority is exercised.

Additionally, during a public health emergency, ASPR can award advanced research and development OTAs expected to cost more than $100 million without a written determination from the HHS Assistant Secretary for Financial Resources. The CARES Act did not provide HHS's National Institutes of Health or DHS with additional OTA flexibilities.

DOD and DHS have established policies requiring the reporting of certain OTAs into FPDS-NG, in part to help address certain statutory reporting requirements.[23] DHS, for example, established policies requiring reporting of research and prototype and Transportation Security Administration OTAs to FPDS-NG.[24] Transportation Security Administration officials stated that they report OTAs to FPDS-NG to also assist with understanding the workload involved in awarding and administering OTAs. HHS ASPR reports its use of OTAs to FPDS-NG while the National Institutes of Health does not.

Overview of Undefinitized Contracts

To help meet urgent needs, agencies can use undefinitized contracts to authorize contractors to begin work and incur costs before reaching final agreement on contract terms and conditions.[25] Before these contracts are

---

[23] The Duncan Hunter National Defense Authorization Act for Fiscal Year 2009 required certain improvements to FPDS-NG, including the collection of data on certain OTAs. Pub. L. No. 110-417, § 874 (2008). DOD does not report its use of research OTAs to FPDS- NG. Instead, DOD requires their use to be reported to the Defense Assistance Awards Data System, a system used to track assistance awards, including grants.

[24] According to DHS officials, DHS requires research and prototype OTAs (issued pursuant to 6 U.S.C. § 391) to be reported in FPDS-NG in accordance with section 874 of the Duncan Hunter National Defense Authorization Act for Fiscal Year 2009. DHS does not require Countering Weapons of Mass Destruction OTAs (issued pursuant to 6 U.S.C. § 596) to be entered into FPDS-NG but still enters these OTAs into FPDS-NG.

[25] For the purposes of our report, we define undefinitized contracts to include letter contracts (a preliminary contract that authorizes the contractor to begin work immediately) pursuant to

finalized, they are called undefinitized. In contrast, a definitized contract is one in which all terms and conditions, including price, are agreed to by the parties to the contract at the time of contract award. We previously found that undefinitized contracts may be risky for the government.[26] In particular, the government may incur unnecessary costs if requirements change before the contract is definitized.

To help minimize these risks:

- The FAR generally requires letter contracts—a type of undefinitized contract—to include a schedule that provides for definitization within 180 days of the contract award or before completion of 40 percent of the work to be performed, whichever occurs first.[27] HHS and DHS are subject to the undefinitized contract requirements in the FAR as well as agency-specific acquisition regulations and policies.
- Additionally, DOD may only enter an undefinitized contract if it requires definitization of the contractual terms, specifications, and price within 180 days of the contractor submitting a qualifying proposal—a proposal that contains sufficient information to enable DOD to conduct meaningful analyses and audits—or before more than 50 percent of the estimated contract price is obligated, whichever occurs first.[28]

FAR § 16.603. In addition, we define undefinitized contracts to include what DOD refers to as "undefinitized contract actions," which includes any contract action for which the contract terms, specifications, or price are not agreed upon before performance has begun under the action. These actions include letters contracts, undefinitized task or delivery orders issued against a pre-established umbrella contract, and undefinitized modifications for additional supplies or services to an existing contract. Defense Federal Acquisition Regulation Supplement subpt. 217.74.

[26] GAO, *Defense Contracting: DOD Has Enhanced Insight into UndefinitizedContract Action Use, but Management at Local Commands Needs Improvement*, GAO-10-299 (Washington, D.C.: Jan. 28, 2010).

[27] FAR § 16.603. For the purposes of our report, we refer to letter contracts as undefinitized contracts.

[28] For the purposes of our report, we refer to the negotiated overall ceiling price and not-to-exceed price in DOD's undefinitized contracts, as well as the proposed estimated cost in HHS's undefinitized contracts, as the estimated contract price. For DOD, if a contractor submits a qualifying proposal to definitize the undefinitized contract before 50 percent of the not-to-exceed price is obligated, the limitation on obligations can be increased to 75 percent of the estimated contract price. 10 U.S.C. § 2326(b) and Defense Federal Acquisition Regulation Supplement subpt. 217.74. See also HHS Acquisition Policy, Guidance and Instructions § 316.603-70.

The CARES Act allows DOD to waive time frames to definitize undefinitized contracts and to waive limitations on the amounts that can be obligated before the undefinitized contract is definitized, which we refer to as CARES Act flexibilities for the purposes of our report.[29] The CARES Act did not provide HHS or DHS with additional flexibilities for undefinitized contracts.

Agencies Obligated at Least $12.5 Billion on OTAs to Quickly Respond to COVID- 19 but Did Not Accurately Report All Awards

DOD, HHS, and DHS obligated at least $12.5 billion on COVID-19-related OTAs from March 2020 through March 2021, primarily to help accelerate vaccine development and manufacturing. However, of that $12.5 billion, at least $1.6 billion was underreported because HHS misreported its OTAs as procurement contracts, while DOD and DHS did not accurately identify certain OTAs as COVID-19-related. In addition, agency officials cited timeliness of award as the main factor contributing to OTA use but also noted that the OTA required less administrative work and facilitated engagement with nontraditional contractors.

Agencies Made Significant Use of OTAs for Vaccine Development and Manufacturing

Our analysis of FPDS-NG and agency-provided data found that DOD, HHS, and DHS obligated at least $12.5 billion on OTAs in response to COVID-19 as of March 2021 (see Figure 1).[30]

These three agencies' obligations on OTAs for COVID-19 have been significant when compared with both of their OTA obligations in prior years and their COVID-19 procurement contract obligations. For example:

---

[29] Pub. L. No. 116-136, § 13005, 134 Stat. at 522.

[30] Prior to March 2020, DHS awarded OTAs in response to COVID-19. These OTAs accounted for $8 million in obligations or 0.07 percent of all COVID-19 OTA obligations and are included in our analysis.

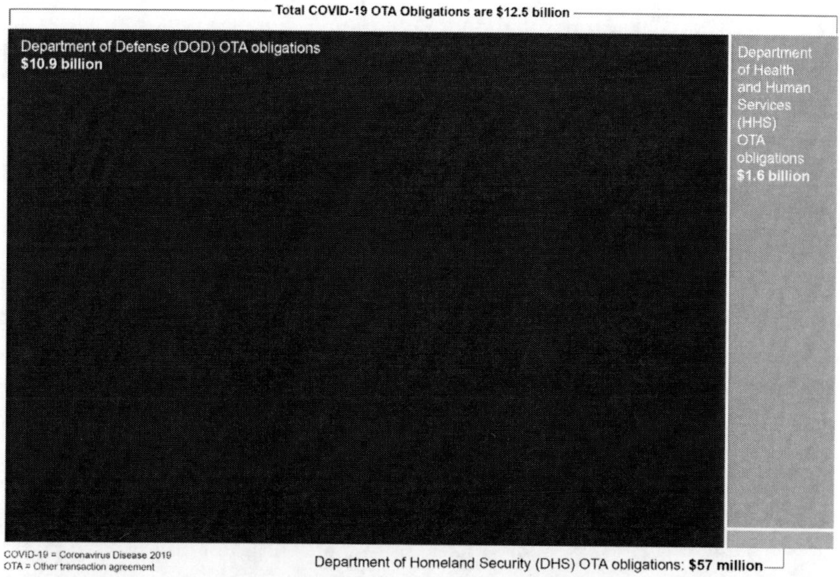
Total COVID-19 OTA Obligations are $12.5 billion
Department of Defense (DOD) OTA obligations
$10.9 billion
Department of Health and Human Services (HHS) OTA obligations
$1.6 billion
COVID-19 = Coronavirus Disease 2019
OTA = Other transaction agreement
Department of Homeland Security (DHS) OTA obligations: $57 million

Source: GAO analysis of Federal Procurement Data System-Next Generation (FPDS-NG) data and information from DOD, HHS, and DHS. | GAO-21-501.

Note: We corrected the FPDS-NG data by adding $1.6 billion in obligations the agencies did not accurately report as COVID-19 OTAs. Our analysis did not include data that are not reported in FPDS-NG because we did not assess the reliability of these data.

Figure 1. DOD, HHS, and DHS Other Transaction Agreement Obligations in Response to Coronavirus Disease 2019 as of March 14, 2021.

- *OTA obligations in prior years.* Obligations reported on OTAs across the three agencies increased from $2.4 billion in fiscal year 2017 to $7.8 billion in fiscal year 2019.[31] In comparison, from March 2020 to March 2021, their OTA obligations were $12.5 billion for the COVID-19 response alone.
- *OTA obligations as a proportion of total obligations.* The three agencies have obligated $54.7 billion in response to COVID-19 using both OTAs and procurement contracts. The $12.5 billion those agencies have obligated on OTAs for COVID-19 represents about 23 percent of the total obligations. In comparison, in fiscal year 2019,

[31] Our fiscal year 2017 through 2019 analysis generally did not include data that are not reported in the FPDS-NG OTA module, such as OTA obligations from the National Institutes of Health, because we did not assess the reliability of these data. However, we supplemented our analysis of FPDS-NG data by including data on OTA obligations provided by HHS ASPR.

prior to the COVID-19 pandemic, their OTA obligations accounted for 2 percent of total obligations.

Of the $12.5 billion obligated on COVID-19 OTAs, $8.9 billion or 71 percent was for vaccine development—including clinical trials—and manufacturing efforts. The remaining $3.6 billion was for medical research and development and other nonvaccine products and services (see Figure 2).

Most of the COVID-19 OTA dollars were obligated in July 2020 and driven by vaccine awards. From November 2020 through March 2021, OTA obligations were comparatively not as significant as earlier in the pandemic, in part because additional vaccine doses were acquired using procurement contracts instead of OTAs (see Figure 3).

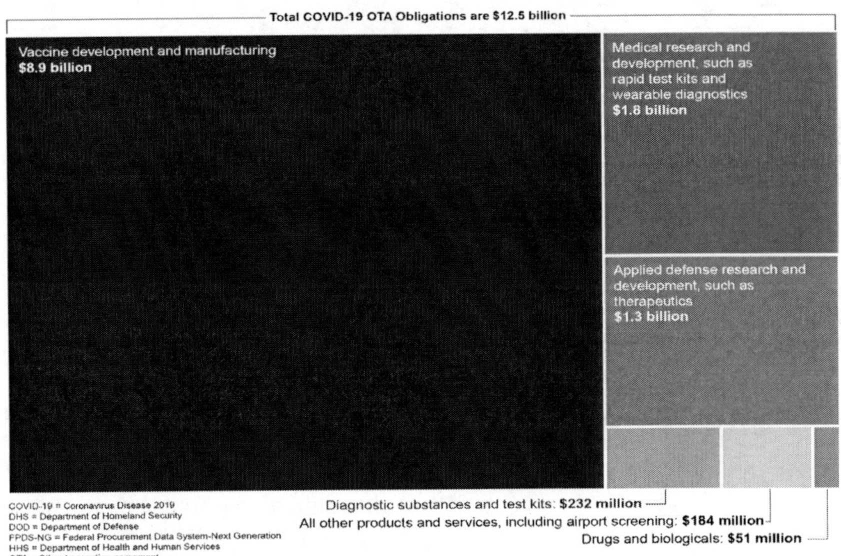

Source: GAO analysis of FPDS-NG data and information from DOD, HHS, and DHS. | GAO-21-501.

Note: We corrected the FPDS-NG data by adding $1.6 billion in obligations the agencies did not accurately report as COVID-19 OTAs. Our analysis did not include data that are not reported in FPDS-NG because we did not assess the reliability of these data.

Figure 2. Top COVID-19 Products and Services Acquired by DOD, HHS, and DHS Using OTAs as of March 14, 2021.

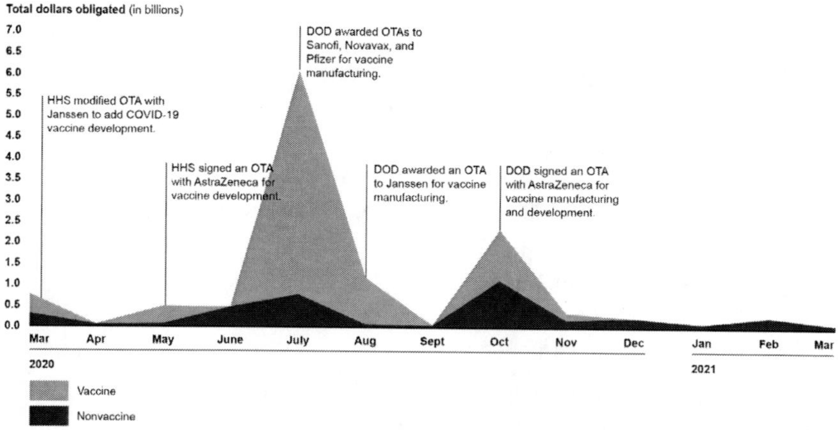

Source: GAO analysis of Federal Procurement Data System-Next Generation (FPDS-NG) data and information from Department of Defense (DOD), Department of Health and Human Services (HHS), and Department of Homeland Security. | GAO-21-501.

Note: We corrected the FPDS-NG data by adding $1.6 billion in obligations the agencies did not accurately report as COVID-19 other transaction agreements (OTA). Our analysis did not include data that are not reported in FPDS-NG because we did not assess the reliability of these data.

Figure 3. Coronavirus Disease 2019 (COVID-19) OTA Obligations by Vaccine and Nonvaccine Awards from March 2020 through March 2021.

Agencies Did Not Accurately Reflect All Dollars Obligated on COVID-19 OTAs

HHS, DOD, and DHS reported obligating $10.9 billion on COVID-19 OTAs in FPDS-NG. However, our analysis of FPDS-NG and agency- provided data, as well as OTA documentation, found these three agencies actually obligated at least $12.5 billion on COVID-19 OTAs—a $1.6 billion difference. In addition to this $1.6 billion, HHS's National Institutes of Health officials told us they obligated about $520 million on COVID-19 OTAs, which were not reported in FPDS-NG.

HHS ASPR was responsible for a majority of the inaccurate reporting of COVID-19 OTA dollars. We previously found in January 2021 that HHS

ASPR misreported its COVID-19 OTAs as procurement contracts because it reports OTAs into the procurement module of FPDS-NG.[32]

Based on our analysis of FPDS-NG data as of March 14, 2021, ASPR continues to misreport these OTAs, which have about $1.55 billion in obligations. ASPR's approach of reporting OTAs in the procurement module is inconsistent with the FAR. Agencies can only report OTAs in FPDS-NG under certain conditions, such as if the OTAs can be segregated from procurement contract actions and written approval from the FPDS program office is obtained.[33] For example, DOD and DHS report certain OTAs in a separate OTA module of FPDS-NG.[34]

Furthermore, ASPR's approach does not provide a way for FPDS-NG users to systematically identify which actions are OTAs. FPDS-NG reflects overreporting of ASPR's COVID-19 procurement contracts by $1.55 billion and no dollars obligated on ASPR's COVID-19 OTAs in the OTA module. In January 2021, we recommended that ASPR should accurately report data in FPDS-NG and provide information that would allow the public to distinguish between spending on OTAs and procurement contracts.[35] ASPR concurred with our recommendation. As of April 2021, ASPR officials stated that they have discussed within ASPR the need to consistently identify OTAs in FPDS-NG and explored how their contract writing system may interface with the FPDS-NG OTA module in the future. ASPR officials added that, in the meantime, they have identified OTAs in the procurement module by manually adding designators such as "OTA" or "other transaction agreement" into the description of requirement data field. We will continue to monitor ASPR's efforts to implement our recommendation.

Separately, DOD and DHS reported their COVID-19 OTAs in the FPDS-NG OTA module but did not accurately identify certain OTAs and associated dollars as COVID-19-related. Specifically:

- In November 2020, DOD obligated $52.5 million on the Pfizer vaccine OTA but did not identify these dollars as COVID-19-related.
- From February 2020 through September 2020, DHS's Countering Weapons of Mass Destruction Office obligated $25.5 million on two

---

[32] GAO-21-265.

[33] FAR § 4.601; 4.603(b); and 4.606(a).

[34] As noted earlier, DOD and DHS are generally not required by statute or regulation to report OTAs into FPDS-NG but have established policies requiring such reporting for certain OTAs.

[35] GAO-21-265.

OTAs for COVID-19 screening at airports and ports of entry but did not identify these OTAs as COVID-19-related.

Additionally, the National Institutes of Health did not report awarding any OTAs in response to COVID-19 in FPDS-NG, as it is not required to do so by statute or policy. In May 2021, National Institutes of Health officials told us they obligated about $520 million on COVID-19 OTAs as of April 2021.[36] Officials told us that while they do not report their use of OTAs to FPDS-NG, they plan to report these OTAs to the Tracking Accountability in Government Grants System—a database used by HHS to track grant awards—starting in summer 2021. Officials stated that such reporting will allow the National Institutes of Health to submit its OTA data to USAspending.gov—a public-facing website that tracks federal spending on procurement and assistance awards. According to officials, the National Institutes of Health has not included information on OTAs in USAspending.gov in the past.

Transparency in federal spending is desired by policymakers and the public. For example, the Federal Funding Accountability and Transparency Act of 2006—which established USAspending.gov—and the Digital Accountability and Transparency Act of 2014 require agencies to disclose spending data on certain federal awards, including contracts and grants.[37] While an agency official—in response to public inquiries on the availability of OTA data on USAspending.gov—noted that the acts are not applicable to OTAs, the Digital Accountability and Transparency Act of 2014 aims to establish government-wide data standards to provide consistent, reliable, and searchable spending data that are displayed accurately for taxpayers and policymakers. Additionally, federal internal control standards state that an agency's management should design information systems and externally communicate quality information to achieve objectives and address related risks.[38]

DOD, DHS, and HHS currently do not use a systematic approach to consistently and accurately track OTAs awarded in response to COVID-19 or other national interest events and the associated dollars obligated. Based on

---

[36] We did not assess the reliability of the data provided by the National Institutes of Health or include them in our analysis.

[37] Pub. L. No. 113-101, 128 Stat. 1146 (May 9, 2014). The Digital Accountability and Transparency Act of 2014 amended the Federal Funding Accountability and Transparency Act of 2006. Pub. L. No. 109-282, 120 Stat. 1186 (Sept. 26, 2006), codified at 31 U.S.C. § 6101 note.

[38] GAO, *Standards for Internal Control in the Federal Government*, GAO-14-704G (Washington, D.C.: September 2014).

our March 2021 analysis, only DOD and DHS reported their COVID-19 OTAs to the FPDS-NG OTA module—a government data system available for agencies to report OTA actions and associated obligations. As noted earlier, while HHS ASPR reported its COVID-19 OTAs to FPDS-NG, it continues to misreport them in the procurement module.

Even if agencies consistently required that their OTA awards be reported to the FPDS-NG OTA module, the module does not have a systematic way for agencies to identify an OTA as COVID-19-related. The procurement contract module of FPDS-NG, in contrast, includes a National Interest Action data field that allows tracking of COVID-19 contracts. According to Office of Management and Budget guidance, National Interest Action codes are used in the procurement module to consistently collect data on contract actions related to emergency or contingency responses or other nationally significant events.[39] Examples of past national interest events tracked by these codes include Hurricanes Katrina, Harvey, Irma, Florence and Michael; Operation Enduring Freedom; and the 2014 Ebola outbreak in West Africa.

In March 2020, GSA added a National Interest Action code to track acquisition costs of federal agencies involved in the response to COVID-19.[40] The Office of Management and Budget later broadened the application of this code, noting that the use of such codes contributes to transparency in tracking of COVID-19-related procurement actions in FPDS-NG.[41] As noted earlier, HHS ASPR continues to misreport its OTAs in the procurement module of FPDS-NG. Because the National Interest Action code data field is available in the procurement module, FPDS-NG users are able to identify which HHS ASPR OTAs are COVID-19-related using this code if ASPR identifies the awards as OTAs in the description of requirement field.

GSA administers the Integrated Award Environment, a government-wide initiative that includes a suite of federal award data systems, including FPDS-NG and its OTA module.[42] According to the Integrated Award Environment's governing charter, the initiative's mission includes simplifying, unifying, and

---

[39] Office of Management and Budget, Office of Federal Procurement Policy, *Memorandum for Chief Acquisition Officers, Senior Procurement Executives: Emergency Acquisitions Guide* (Washington, D.C.: Jan. 14, 2011).

[40] Office of Management and Budget, *Memorandum to the Heads of Executive Departments and Agencies: Managing Federal Contract Performance Issues Associated with the Novel Coronavirus (COVID-19)*, M-20-18 (Washington, D.C.: Mar. 20, 2020).

[41] Office of Management and Budget, *Memorandum for the Heads of Departments and Agencies: Implementation Guidance for Supplemental Funding Provided in Response to the Coronavirus Disease 2019 (COVID-19)*, M-20-21 (Washington, D.C.: Apr. 10, 2020).

[42] The Integrated Award Environment is a GSA-managed presidential e-government initiative established in 2002.

streamlining the federal award process for government agencies, which it achieves through changes to a portfolio of government-wide online systems. The initiative has a change control board, which includes 24 voting members from agencies identified in the Chief Financial Officer Act—including DOD, DHS, HHS, and GSA. Any revisions to FPDS-NG must be approved by a majority of the agencies that are voting members.

According to GSA officials, as of April 2021, no agency requested to add the National Interest Action data element to the OTA module. GSA officials explained that not all of the agencies use the OTA module. However, because updates to the FPDS-NG system and other Integrated Award Environment systems are collectively funded by all 24 agencies, each agency has a vote in how the funding is spent and what system changes are prioritized. GSA is currently leading an effort to modernize the Integrated Award Environment systems, including FPDS-NG, which may offer an alternative system and process for reporting on OTAs. However, GSA officials did not have time frames for when the new system will be implemented.

Adding a National Interest Action data field to the OTA module is one option for tracking OTAs used for national emergencies such as the pandemic response. Without this or another systematic approach, policy makers and the public will continue to lack insight into the extent to which agencies are using OTAs to respond to national emergencies.

Additionally, due to a lack of a systematic way to identify national interest events for OTA awards, agencies take different approaches over how and whether they distinguish COVID-19 OTAs from other OTAs. In March 2020, DOD issued guidance informing contracting personnel that the OTA module does not have a National Interest Action data field and instructed them to enter "COVID-19" in the description of requirement data field.[43]

DHS, however, does not have guidance on how COVID-19 OTAs should be specifically identified in the OTA module. While DHS's March 2020 National Interest Action code guidance emphasizes the importance of all DHS-related FPDS-NG actions being promptly and correctly coded as COVID-19 for congressional oversight, it does not include information on how OTAs should be specifically coded.[44] Without such guidance, public

---

[43] Department of Defense, Office of the Under Secretary of Defense for Acquisition and Sustainment, *Reporting COVID-19 Related Actions to the Federal Procurement Data System* (Washington, D.C.: Mar. 31, 2020).

[44] Department of Homeland Security, Chief Procurement Officer, *Increasing Thresholds for Procurements Supporting Coronavirus (COVID-19) Response and Recovery* (Washington, D.C.: Mar. 17, 2020).

users of FPDS-NG will not have an accurate understanding of the extent to which DHS used OTAs in response to COVID-19.

Timeliness among Top Factors Cited for OTA Use in Response to COVID-19

DOD and HHS Used OTAs to Help Expedite Large Vaccine Awards

DOD and HHS officials cited the timeliness of awards as one of the main factors for using OTAs for COVID-19 vaccine development and manufacturing. Vaccine development efforts included clinical trials that evaluated the product's safety, efficacy, proposed doses, schedule of immunizations, and methods of delivery in volunteers. Vaccine manufacturing efforts included large-scale production of hundreds of millions of doses that met the Food and Drug Administration's regulatory standards for ensuring pharmaceutical quality. According to OTA justification documents and DOD officials, OTAs offered streamlined competitive processes for evaluation and selection of awardees. Seven OTAs awarded by either HHS or DOD accounted for all $8.9 billion in OTA obligations on vaccine development and manufacturing (see Table 1).

More broadly, OTAs have played a significant role in the joint effort between DOD and HHS to expedite the acquisition and development of COVID-19 vaccine candidates—previously known as the Operation Warp Speed effort.[45] For example, the seven vaccine OTAs we reviewed accounted for 43 percent of the $20.5 billion obligated by DOD and HHS on vaccine development and manufacturing as of March 14, 2021.[46]

The award times for the COVID-19 vaccine OTAs were generally shorter than award times for OTAs and procurement contracts we reviewed in our prior work in 2018 and 2019. We defined award times as the time from the contracting office releasing a solicitation until the time the government awarded the OTA. Specifically, for the six vaccine OTAs awarded in response to a COVID-19 solicitation, the award times ranged from 27 days to about 8

---

[45] As of January 20, 2021, the federal government no longer uses the name Operation Warp Speed, but the DOD and HHS partnership has continued. DOD and HHS's partnership was formalized through a memorandum of understanding between the two departments. For more information on COVID-19 vaccines, see GAO-21-443.

[46] The remaining $11.4 billion in obligations were on contract vehicles outside the scope of this review. For example, these vehicles included $5.3 billion in procurement contracts awarded to Moderna for vaccine development.

months, with a median of 54 days.[47] For non-COVID-19 OTAs, in November 2019, we found that award times for a nongeneralizable sample of 11 DOD prototype OTAs ranged from 45 days to about 1 year, with a median of nearly 10 months.[48] For procurement contracts, in July 2018, we found that the award time for 129 weapon systems-related contracts ranged from less than a month to over 4 years, with a median of about 9 months.[49]

Table 1. Dollars obligated on OTAs awarded by DOD and HHS for COVID-19 vaccine development and manufacturing by manufacturer as of March 14, 2021

Contracting agency	Vaccine manufacturer (effort)	Total dollars obligated ($)
HHS ASPR	Janssen (development and clinical studies)	1.1 billion
DOD Army	Janssen (manufacturing)	1.0 billion
HHS ASPR	AstraZeneca (development)	0.126 billion
DOD Army	AstraZeneca (manufacturing)	1.2 billion
DOD Army	Sanofi (manufacturing)	1.8 billion
DOD Army	Novavax (manufacturing)	1.6 billion
DOD Army	Pfizer (manufacturing)	2.03 billion
Total		8.9 billion

ASPR - Office of the Assistant Secretary for Preparedness and Response
COVID-19 - Coronavirus Disease 2019
DOD - Department of Defense
FPDS - NG - Federal Procurement Data System-Next Generation
HHS - Department of Health and Human Services
OTA - Other transaction agreement
Source: GAO analysis of FPDS-NG data and information from DOD and HHS. | GAO-21-501.
Note: We corrected the FPDS-NG data by adding $1.3 billion in obligations the agencies did not accurately report as COVID-19 OTAs. Our analysis did not include data that are not reported in FPDS-NG because we did not assess the reliability of these data.

DOD and HHS employed several contracting methods to further expedite the award of the seven vaccine OTAs (see Table 2).

[47] We excluded from our analysis of award times the ASPR-awarded OTA to Janssen because it was awarded prior to the COVID-19 pandemic. The six OTAs included in our analysis were five awarded by Army Contracting Command to Janssen, Sanofi, Novavax, Pfizer, and AstraZeneca, and one awarded by ASPR to AstraZeneca. Both of the AstraZeneca OTAs—one awarded in May 2020 and the other in October 2020—were in response to the same solicitation issued in March 2020.

[48] GAO-20-84.

[49] GAO, *Defense Contracts: DOD Should Develop a Strategy for Assessing Contract Award Time Frames*, GAO-18-467 (Washington, D.C.: July 16, 2018).

Table 2. Methods used by DOD and HHS in awarding OTAs to help expedite COVID-19 vaccine development and manufacturing

Methods to expedite award of OTAs	Contracting agency/vaccine manufacturer						
	Army/ Janssen	HHS ASPR/ Janssen	Army/ AstraZeneca	HHS ASPR/ AstraZeneca	Army/ Sanofi	Army/ Novavax	Army/ Pfizer
DOD and HHS partnership	✓	✗	✓	✗	✓	✓	✓
DOD OTA award that continues work of previously awarded HHS OTA	✓	✗	✓[a]	✗[a]	✗	✗	✗
Modified existing OTA to add projects	✓	✓	✗	✗	✓	✓	✓
Awarded OTAs without finalized terms and conditions	✗	✗	✓	✓	✓	✓	✗
Delegated approval to lower-level management review pursuant to the CARES Act	✓	✗	✓	✗	✓	✓	✓
Congressional notification requirement not provided in advance pursuant to the CARES Act	✓	✗	✓	✗	✓	✓	✓

Legend:

✓ = yes

✗ = no or not applicable

ASPR - Office of the Assistant Secretary for Preparedness and Response

COVID-19 - Coronavirus Disease 2019

DOD - Department of Defense

HHS - Department of Health and Human Services

OTA - other transaction agreement

Source: GAO analysis of DOD and HHS OTA documentation and testimonial information from officials. | GAO-21-501

[a]Army officials stated that their October 2020 OTA award to AstraZeneca replaced and finalized the OTA that HHS ASPR had awarded in May 2020.

The methods used by DOD and HHS to expedite vaccine development and manufacturing in their OTA awards are further illustrated below:

- *DOD and HHS partnership.* According to DOD and HHS officials, HHS partnered with DOD to leverage DOD's OTA authorities and acquisition workforce capacity, which HHS lacked. First, HHS ASPR's OTA authority is limited to advanced research and development, while DOD's OTA authority allows for research, prototyping, and production efforts. However, while DOD awarded five vaccine prototype OTAs, it did not award any follow-on vaccine production OTAs as of March 2021. For example, to acquire an additional 200 million Pfizer vaccine doses after the initial 100 million acquired under the prototype OTA, DOD awarded $4 billion in procurement contracts. DOD officials explained that, when they began negotiating the follow-on contracts with Pfizer for additional doses in December 2020, Pfizer had not yet fully demonstrated its prototyping efforts under the OTA—namely, delivering 100 million doses. Successful prototype project completion is one of the conditions that must be met to award a follow-on production OTA without being required to use competitive procedures.[1]
  Second, according to senior HHS contracting officials, the contracting needs resulting from COVID-19 overwhelmed HHS's acquisition workforce both in terms of capacity and expertise. In March 2021, a third-party company assessed the office of HHS's senior procurement executive and found the office does not have sufficient staffing.
  Additionally, the assessment noted that the office had limited funding for acquisition staffing and did not provide sufficient oversight of contracts and the acquisition workforce. Further, the assessment found HHS had outdated contracting policies.
- *DOD OTA awards that continue work of previously-awarded HHS OTAs.* As part of the DOD and HHS partnership, Army Contracting Command awarded OTAs that continued COVID-19 work started under OTAs awarded by ASPR. For example, in May 2020, ASPR awarded AstraZeneca an OTA for vaccine development without finalized terms and conditions, in anticipation of another OTA award that would replace it. In October 2020, Army Contracting Command

[1] 10 U.S.C. 2371b(f)(2)(B).

awarded a $1.2 billion prototype OTA that built upon AstraZeneca's efforts in developing and manufacturing the vaccine under ASPR's OTA. After Army Contracting Command awarded the OTA to AstraZeneca, ASPR terminated its OTA, which had $126 million in obligations.

- *DOD and HHS modified existing OTAs to add projects.* For four of the vaccine OTAs, Army Contracting Command modified an existing OTA for COVID-19 prototype projects awarded to Janssen, Sanofi, Novavax, and Pfizer.[2] ASPR also modified an OTA previously awarded to Janssen to include COVID-19 vaccine development in the scope. A senior ASPR official explained that Janssen's existing OTA provided HHS with the flexibility to quickly pivot from an existing portfolio of vaccines to focus on COVID-19, which would not have been possible under a procurement contract.
- *DOD and HHS awarded OTAs without finalized terms and conditions.* In July and October 2020, Army Contracting Command made vaccine awards to Sanofi, Novavax, and AstraZeneca that were not finalized. DOD senior contracting officials stated that doing so allowed the vaccine manufacturers to initiate work quickly. According to Army Contracting Command officials, examples of terms and conditions not finalized included the total project costs and elements of project scope, including the clinical trials. According to officials, all three OTAs were finalized in December 2020, 2 to 5 months after the awards. As noted earlier, ASPR also awarded an OTA to AstraZeneca without finalized terms and conditions, such as what intellectual property rights the government would receive. ASPR officials stated that this approach allowed AstraZeneca to initiate work quickly.
- *DOD used CARES Act flexibility to delegate approval of OTAs to lower-level management review.* Of the six vaccine OTAs that met the dollar thresholds to use CARES Act flexibilities for the initial award, five used the flexibility that allowed lower-level contracting officials to approve the OTAs.[3] Specifically, the Army's senior procurement executive, rather than the Under Secretary of Defense for Research and Engineering or the Under Secretary of Defense for

[2] Janssen is a pharmaceutical subsidiary of Johnson & Johnson.

[3] ASPR awarded an OTA to Janssen in August 2017, prior to passage of the CARES Act in March 2020. The CARES Act flexibility was not used for the initial award. Pub. L. No. 116-136, § 3301.

Acquisition and Sustainment, approved the written determinations for these five OTAs.[4]

- *DOD used CARES Act flexibility to provide congressional notifications after awards.* All five vaccine OTAs awarded by DOD used the CARES flexibility to notify the congressional defense committees in writing of these OTAs after they were awarded (rather than the typical requirement of notification at least 30 days before award).[5] For all five vaccine OTAs, DOD notified the committees within 1 week of award.

Additionally, the written justifications for four of the vaccine OTAs cited the flexibility to negotiate individualized OTA language and unique terms and conditions that would not have been possible under a procurement contract as factors contributing to the use of OTAs. For example, DOD officials cited flexible payment terms through milestone payment schedules, flexible termination provisions, and custom rights for intellectual property, technical data, and regulatory deliverables.

DOD, HHS, and DHS Cited Timeliness and Other Factors for Nonvaccine OTAs

Factors that contributed to agencies using OTAs for the eight selected nonvaccine efforts included (1) timeliness of awards, (2) a more flexible process which requires less administrative work, (3) engaging nontraditional contractors, and (4) the ability to use cost-sharing or additional funding streams (see Table 3).

The factors that contributed to the use of OTAs are further illustrated in the examples below.

- *Timeliness of awards.* Contracting officials noted that the OTAs allowed them to successfully execute efforts in weeks, whereas a procurement contract would generally take months to award.[6] For example, in February 2020, the DHS Countering Weapons of Mass

[4] The five OTAs that met the $500 million estimated cost threshold and used the CARES Act flexibility related to approval delegation from the Under Secretary of Defense for Research and Engineering or the Under Secretary of Defense for Acquisition and Sustainment to other officials for prototype OTAs were the Janssen, AstraZeneca, Pfizer, Novavax, and Sanofi OTAs.

[5] Pub. L. No. 116-136, § 13006(b).

[6] DOD and Transportation Security Administration officials stated that OTA awards are not always faster to award than procurement contracts.

Destruction Office noncompetitively awarded a $23 million OTA for COVID-19 screening at airports and ports of entry within 1 day of receiving the requirement. DHS officials stated that the contractor began work based on a verbal agreement and then signed a written OTA award 24 days later. In another example, ASPR's approval document for an OTA awarded to Regeneron for therapeutics against emerging infectious diseases noted significant time savings as a benefit of using OTAs. According to the approval document, the OTA allowed for the immediate replacement of underperforming assets within a therapeutics portfolio with a promising new candidate, which resulted in an estimated savings of up to 9 months and hundreds of hours of government effort. ASPR officials explained that under a procurement contract, terminating work and adding scope can take longer given the additional FAR requirements that must be met to do so, such as those related to terminations or competition for modifications that change the scope of work.

- *More flexible contracting process and less administrative work.* According to officials interviewed and the approval documents for all eight OTAs we reviewed, OTAs have a more flexible process and require less administrative work than procurement contracts. For example, in April 2020, Army Contracting Command modified an existing production OTA for a suite of communication capabilities used in national emergencies to include $11 million for use of such capabilities at COVID-19 testing sites.[7] Army Contracting Command officials noted that these OTAs required less administrative work to execute, including less required documentation than a procurement contract.

[7] Army Contracting Command officials awarded this production OTA to Augustine Consulting, Inc. upon the successful completion of their prototype under a separate prototype OTA. According to FPDS-NG data as of October 2020, this OTA was the only production OTA awarded by DOD, which in part covered some of the communications equipment used for the COVID-19 response.

Table 3. Cited benefits of using OTAs for selected nonvaccine COVID-19 efforts cited by DOD, HHS, and DHS

Cited Benefits of OTAs	Nonvaccine OTA							
	Army crisis response technology	Army rapid test kits	Army wearable COVID-19 detection	Army Regeneron therapeutic	HHS ASPR Regeneron therapeutic	Air Force 3D printing	DHS airport and port screening	DHS airport cleaning
Timeliness of awards	✓	✓	✓	✓	✓	✗	✓	✓
More flexible process or less administrative work	✓	✓	✓	✓	✓	✓	✓	✓
Nontraditional contractor engagement	✓	✓	✓	✓	✓	✓	✓	✓
Cost-sharing or use of additional funding streams	✗	✗	✗	✗	✓	✓	✗	✗

Legend:
✓ = yes
✗ = no or not applicable
ASPR - Office of the Assistant Secretary for Preparedness and Response
COVID-19 - Coronavirus Disease 2019
DHS - Department of Homeland Security
DOD - Department of Defense
HHS - Department of Health and Human Services
OTA - Other transaction agreement
Source: GAO analysis of DOD and HHS OTA documentation and testimonial information from officials. | GAO-21-501.

- *Nontraditional contractor engagement.* Most of the nonvaccine OTAs in our review were awarded to nontraditional contractors. For example, in August and September 2020, the Army Medical Research Acquisition Activity awarded OTAs with combined total obligations of $19.2 million for seven nontraditional contractors to develop COVID-19 wearable diagnostic devices. Army Medical Research Acquisition Activity officials told us the OTAs enabled them to engage with commercial companies that do not normally do business with DOD. One such example is Fitbit. Army officials stated that military work does not typically fit into Fitbit's business model, but it entered into an OTA for diagnostic devices. Similarly, HHS officials stated that many biomedical research and development organizations are unable or unwilling to agree to some government conditions in procurement contracts, which they perceive to be burdensome.

In another example, in October 2020, Army Contracting Command awarded a $481 million OTA to Cue Inc. for rapid COVID-19 detection testing kits, which were the official test kits for the National Basketball Association. Army Contracting Command officials told us that the OTA provided a collaborative "training wheels" type of arrangement. This allowed Cue Inc. to learn how to be a government contractor and allowed the government to learn how to use Cue Inc.'s new technology, which would not have been possible under a traditional contracting mechanism.

- *OTAs allowed for cost-sharing and ability to use additional funding streams.* Cost-sharing on an OTA occurs when a portion of the total cost is paid by sources other than the federal government. For example, in September 2020, the Air Force awarded an OTA with $4.3 million in obligations to Essentium Inc. that was used to support the defense industrial base for 3D printing capabilities. The Air Force plans to leverage this 3D printing capability to address maintenance and obsolescence issues in aircraft. In April 2021, we found that COVID-19 exacerbated challenges at Air Force depots, such as having too few materials to finish work.[8]

  Air Force officials explained that this OTA award helped increase cash flow to the contractor to offset financial distress caused by COVID-19. The Air Force awarded this OTA through a small business innovation research pilot program, which has a cost-sharing requirement.
- Specifically, the program has a matching-funds requirement: For every dollar of small business innovation research funding provided, nonfederal sources must fund one dollar, and a private third-party must fund two dollars. Air Force officials stated that accommodating this cost-sharing requirement was a fundamental reason and benefit for using an OTA for the effort.

[8] GAO, *Depot Maintenance: DOD Should Improve Pandemic Plans and Publish Working Capital Fund Policy*, GAO-21-103 (Washington, D.C.: Apr. 6, 2021).

Similar to the vaccine OTAs, two of the nonvaccine OTAs—Army Contracting Command's Regeneron therapeutics and COVID-19 rapid test kit OTAs—used the CARES Act flexibility to delegate approval to lower-level management reviews.[9] The Army's head of contracting activity—rather than the senior procurement executive—approved the written determinations for both OTAs. Five nonvaccine OTAs we reviewed did not use the CARES Act flexibility because they were (1) awarded by DHS, which did not receive OTA flexibilities under the CARES Act; or (2) below the relevant dollar thresholds. The remaining nonvaccine OTA was awarded prior to the flexibilities being granted.

Majority of COVID-19 OTA Obligations Awarded through Consortia, but Transparency and Oversight Are Limited

DOD awarded about 58 percent of the $12.5 billion in COVID-19 OTA obligations to members of consortia through a single consortium management firm, but agencies did not report which members received the awards and do not have policies that address the need for enhanced oversight of firm-managed consortia OTAs. DOD, HHS, and DHS did not publicly report which consortium members received OTA awards because of limitations with FPDS-NG, which reduces the transparency of these OTAs. In addition, consortium management firms can provide acquisition- support services for OTA awards that require heightened management attention from the government. However, DOD and HHS policies do not address mitigation of this known risk.

$7.2 Billion of OTA Obligations Awarded through One Consortium Management Firm

According to FPDS-NG, the top recipient of COVID-19 OTA obligations was Advanced Technology International (ATI), a consortium management firm (see Figure 4).[10]

---

[9] These two OTAs met the $100 million cost threshold to use DOD's CARES Act flexibility related to the senior procurement executives delegating approval of written determinations to other officials. Pub. L. No. 116-136, § 13006(a).

[10] According to its website, ATI manages 21 different consortia—15 through OTAs and six through procurement contracts.

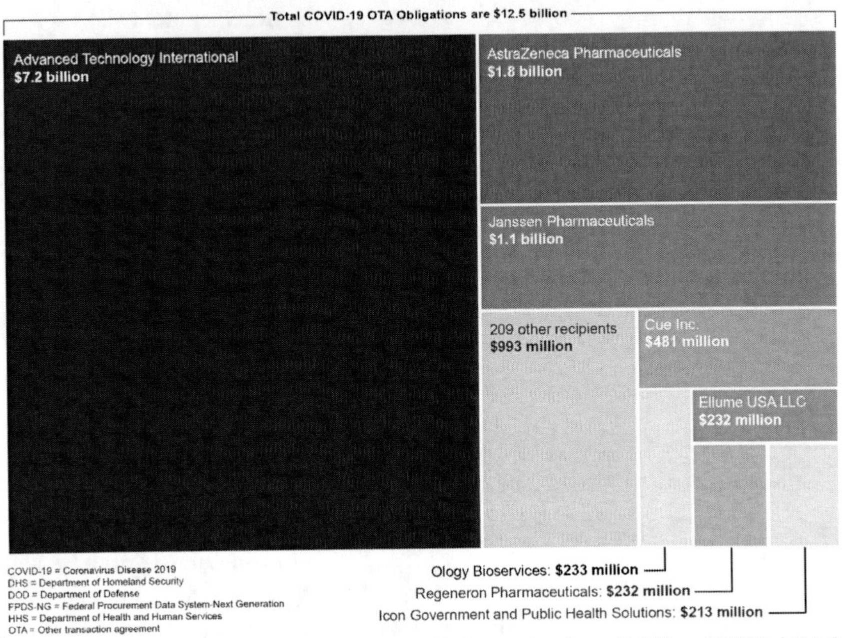

Source: GAO analysis of FPDS-NG data and information from DOD and HHS. | GAO-21-501.

Note: We corrected the FPDS-NG data by adding $1.6 billion in obligations the agencies did not accurately report as COVID-19 OTAs. Our analysis did not include data that are not reported in FPDS-NG because we did not assess the reliability of these data.

Figure 4. Top Recipients of COVID-19 OTA Obligations as of March 14, 2021.

Prior to the COVID-19 response, OTA awards to ATI accounted for $3.5 billion, or 49 percent of the obligations on DOD's prototype OTA awards from fiscal years 2016 through 2018.[11]

A consortium is comprised of members which can include traditional contractors, nontraditional companies, nonprofit organizations, and academic institutions interested in a specific topic area. A consortium can be established to provide the government a pool of stakeholders to further innovate in that topic area. According to ATI staff, some of these consortium members may be less experienced in contracting with the government. A consortium management firm may administratively manage the consortium and act as a liaison or broker between the members and the government in OTA awards (see Figure 5).

---

[11] GAO-20-84.

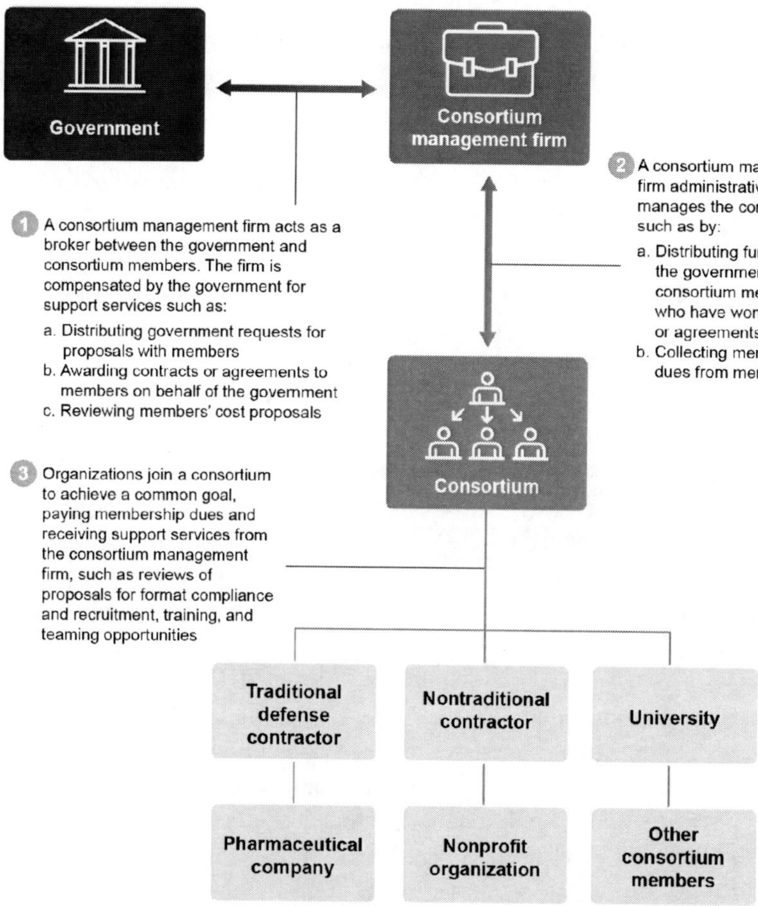

Source: GAO analysis of Department of Defense information and Advanced Technology International (data); iiierlok_xolms/stock.adobe.com (images). | GAO-21-501.

Figure 5. Notional Depiction of Relationships for One Type of Consortium Other Transaction Agreement Model.

As a consortium management firm, ATI manages multiple consortia. ATI provides administrative support services that facilitate the contracting process and does not perform prototype or production work under OTAs. For example, ATI receives requests for prototype proposals from DOD and distributes them to consortium members through an ATI-managed solicitation system. ATI then reviews consortium members' proposals to ensure all required documentation is complete before submitting it to DOD. ATI, on behalf of the consortia, also negotiates the terms and conditions of base or "umbrella" OTA awards between DOD and consortium members when such an approach is used. The base OTA provides terms and conditions that generally apply to all project OTAs awarded and serves as a starting point for negotiations between DOD and consortium member awardees. For the six OTAs awarded through ATI in our review, DOD paid ATI for its services under a cost-plus-fixed-fee structure to assist in executing OTAs, which include acquisition support services. Separately, consortium members pay dues to the consortium.

For the COVID-19 response, three consortia managed by ATI have received OTA awards: the Medical Chemical, Biological, Radiological and Nuclear Defense Consortium (hereafter referred to as the medical defense consortium), the Medical Technology Enterprise Consortium (hereafter referred to as the medical technology consortium), and the Countering Weapons of Mass Destruction Consortium.[12] According to DOD and ASPR officials, awarding OTAs to consortia provided two main benefits to the government for responding to COVID-19: a ready supply of organizations interested in the subject matter and faster negotiation times due to streamlined solicitation and selection procedures. For example:

- *Medical defense consortium.* In April 2016, Army Contracting Command awarded a 20-year base OTA with an estimated ceiling of $10 billion to the medical defense consortium through ATI. This OTA was for conducting research and development into medical, pharmaceutical, and diagnostic technologies to enhance mission effectiveness of military personnel. From this base OTA, Army Contracting Command awarded four vaccine OTAs and one therapeutic OTA. According to DOD officials, the base OTA's terms and conditions provided a starting point for negotiations, which expedited the negotiation process. The average award time for the five medical defense consortium OTAs was 45 days.
- *Medical technology consortium.* In August 2015, Army Medical Research Acquisition Activity awarded a 10-year base OTA to ATI to help establish a medical technology consortium that could perform on future OTA projects.[13] The projects include conducting research, development, and testing leading to technology demonstrations in the biomedical sciences and related fields to maintain and improve service member health and performance. Army Medical Research

[12] ATI waived its fixed fee for all COVID-19 awards.

[13] According to ATI officials, after the medical technology consortium was established as a legal entity, the OTA was novated or transferred to the consortium on August 31, 2016.

> Acquisition Activity officials explained that the OTA consortium model allows them to engage with medical companies that are not accustomed to and generally do not want to navigate the government procurement process. These officials also stated that ATI can rapidly distribute their government solicitations to a pool of more than 300 medical technology consortium members that are already aware of or engaged in work compatible with the activity's needs.

Additionally, ASPR officials stated that while they previously did not award many OTAs to consortia, they were interested in expanding their use as a result of their positive experience with DOD and the medical defense consortium. Specifically, ASPR officials stated that consortia provide a ready pool of companies to respond to requests for proposals.

Agencies Generally Do Not Report Data on Consortium Members Receiving OTA Awards

When federal agencies award OTAs to consortia, they do not report which consortia members received the awards because the OTA module of FPDS-NG does not currently have the capability to allow for this reporting. Instead, the OTA module tracks the top-level awardee—the consortium or consortium management firm—but is opaque beyond that. For example, our analysis of FPDS-NG data showed ATI receiving $7.2 billion in OTA obligations in response to COVID-19. However, our analysis of OTA award documentation, publicly available data, and data provided by ATI found that the majority of that funding was distributed to five OTA awardees who performed the work. ATI received about 0.12 percent of the obligations to fund its support services (see Figure 6).

In another example, analysis of FPDS-NG data showed the medical technology consortium—which is managed by ATI—received $19.2 million for the wearable COVID-19 diagnostics OTA award. Our analysis of OTA documents for this project found that seven nontraditional defense contractors—the University of California, San Francisco; Diomics; Silbel; Philips; Empatica; Sempulse; and Fitbit—each received from $1.8 million to $5.2 million to perform the work.[14] The medical technology consortium and

[14] The request for prototype proposal for this OTA was open to both members and nonmembers of the medical technology consortium. The request for prototype proposals further noted that,

ATI did not receive any of the $19.2 million. Instead, ATI received a separate payment of about $885,000 to reimburse OTA-execution costs, which was awarded under the base OTA and not identified as COVID-19-related.

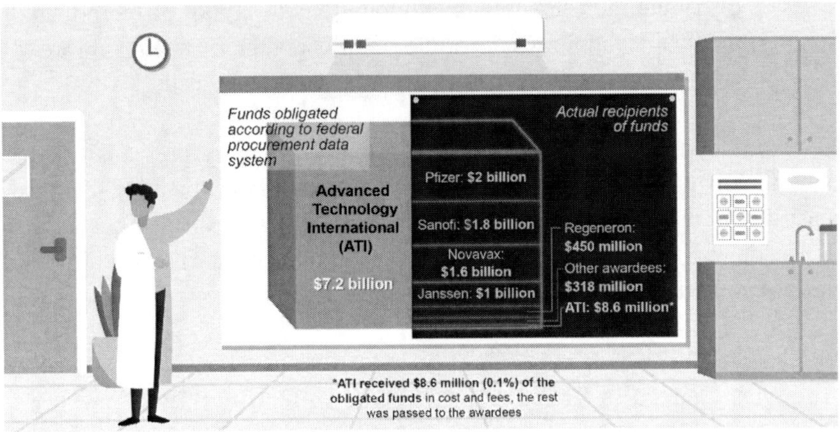

Source: GAO analysis of Federal Procurement Data System-Next Generation data, data and other transaction agreement documents from the Department of Defense, and data from Advanced Technology International. (data); djvstock/stock.adobe.com (doctor image). | GAO-21-501.

Figure 6. Coronavirus Disease 19 Other Transaction Agreement Awardees and Obligations in Federal Procurement Database Compared to Awardees Who Actually Received Funds as of March 14, 2021.

ATI staff told us that the FPDS-NG OTA data overstate how much ATI has received, making it appear that ATI retains billions in funding for its services. ATI staff stated that the way the government reports OTA data into FPDS-NG does not accurately capture ATI's role. For the OTAs awarded through ATI, the government selects which consortium members receive awards and the amount of those awards. To this end, ATI's consortia websites provide some information on the consortium members who received awards and the amounts each member received by solicitation.

In November 2019, we found similar OTA data system limitations, and DOD officials at that time stated they were working to address them.[15] In April

if a nonmember submitted a proposal that was selected by the government, the nonmember was required to join the consortium to receive an OTA award. The medical technology consortium is administratively managed by ATI but is separately identified in FPDS-NG, unlike the medical defense consortium.

[15] GAO-20-84.

2021, the DOD Inspector General also found that FPDS-NG did not provide insight into consortium member awardees for non-COVID-19 OTAs awarded through consortia, among other data limitations.[16] The DOD Inspector General recommended that DOD coordinate with GSA to update FPDS-NG to more accurately capture data related to OTAs awarded through consortia. DOD concurred with the recommendation and stated that it was requesting FPDS-NG updates through the Integrated Award Environment.

In April 2021, DOD officials told us they were proposing two changes to the OTA module—one that would allow tracking of whether an OTA was awarded to a consortium or not and one that would allow tracking of which consortium members performed work on the OTA. However, DOD officials added that they face challenges implementing changes related to adding the capability to track consortium members. One challenge is that FPDS-NG changes are resource-constrained and must be prioritized by a majority of the Integrated Award Environment governing board. As noted earlier, the board includes DOD, DHS, HHS, and GSA. Another issue is that more broadly, GSA is leading an effort to revamp how federal contractors are identified and tracked, which is to be completed by April 2022. DOD officials explained that they may wait until this tracking effort is implemented before adding the capability to track consortium member awardees for OTAs. While DOD's proposed changes to the FPDS-NG OTA module could provide the necessary insight into consortium member awardees, these changes may not be prioritized by the Integrated Award Environment given other competing demands for FPDS-NG and other system changes.

Until the agencies have the capability to systematically track the consortium members who received OTAs, information on the consortium member awardees could be included in the description of requirement field in the OTA module. As of April 2021, DOD, HHS, and DHS indicated they have not required agreement officers to do so.

Additionally, agencies do not consistently provide this type of information to congressional decision makers. For example, DOD's fiscal year 2019 report on the use of OTAs submitted to the congressional defense committees includes information on whether OTAs were awarded to a consortium but does not include information on the consortium member awardees.[17] In contrast,

---

[16] Department of Defense Inspector General, *Audit of Other Transactions Awarded Through Consortiums*, DODIG-2021-077 (Alexandria, VA: Apr. 21, 2021).

[17] Department of Defense, Office of the Under Secretary of Defense for Acquisition and Sustainment, *Report to Congress on the Use of Other Transactions (OT) Authority for*

DHS's fiscal year 2019 report on OTAs submitted to the congressional homeland security committees includes some information on consortium members who received OTA awards.[18] However, DHS's OTA reports are not published, so taxpayers do not have insight into which consortium members have received OTA awards from DHS. According to HHS officials, HHS did not have a requirement to report on its OTA use to congressional committees prior to the pandemic and thus also has not provided OTA consortia awardee information to congressional decision makers.[19]

According to DOD, HHS, and DHS policies, one of the primary objectives of agencies for using OTAs is to build new relationships with entities that may not ordinarily do business with the government, such as start-up companies. Further, federal standards for internal controls state that an agency's management should externally communicate quality information to achieve its objectives and related risks.[20]

Without transparency on the awardees who are performing the work on OTAs awarded to consortia, congressional decision makers and taxpayers have limited insight into the extent to which agencies are achieving one of the purposes of awarding OTAs—attracting nontraditional contractors.

DOD and HHS Policies Do Not Address Risks for Consortium OTAs That Need Heightened Management Attention

When consortium management firms perform acquisition-support services—activities that closely support inherently governmental functions—they often require heightened management attention. For all six OTAs that DOD awarded through ATI in our review, documentation of DOD's analysis of risks or mitigation steps related to this heightened attention was lacking.

According to the Office of Federal Procurement Policy's Policy Letter 11-01, inherently governmental functions refer to functions that are so intimately related to the public interest, they are required to be performed by federal

---

Prototype Projects in FY 2019 and First Quarter of FY 2020 (Washington, D.C.: Apr. 16, 2020).

[18] Department of Homeland Security, Office of the Chief Procurement Officer, *Other Transaction Authority, Fiscal Year 2019* (Washington, D.C.: Nov. 4, 2020).

[19] The CARES Act requires HHS to provide a report to the certain congressional committees on the funds used for OTAs using certain CARES Act flexibilities after expiration of the public health emergency declaration. Pub. L. No. 116-136, §§ 3301.

[20] GAO-14-704G.

employees.[21] One example of such a function is the determination of whether prices are fair and reasonable when awarding contracts. Additionally, the policy letter identifies categories of service functions that are not considered inherently governmental and that agencies are allowed to contract for but that require heightened management attention because they are closely associated with the performance of inherently governmental functions. These types of service functions may require enhanced attention because of the possibility that contractors may inappropriately influence the government's authority, control, and accountability for decisions.

According to the policy letter, an agency can determine that contractor performance of such a service function is appropriate. However, for all procurements of services above the simplified acquisition threshold where the contracted function is closely associated with an inherently governmental function, the agency should identify—during the acquisition planning phase—risk mitigation steps to oversee and manage the contractor's activities.[22] Specifically, the agency should document in the contract file an analysis that establishes that the agency has sufficient capacity and capability to give special management attention to contractor performance and limit or guide the contractor's discretion, among other analyses.

As noted earlier, consortium management firms such as ATI can provide acquisition-support services to the government that closely support inherently governmental functions. For the six consortium OTAs in our review, ATI's acquisition-support responsibilities are outlined in the terms and conditions of the base OTAs, which generally apply to the OTAs awarded to consortia members. ATI's acquisition-support responsibilities for the COVID-19 wearable diagnostic devices OTA are outlined in the terms and conditions associated with the August 2015 base OTA awarded to the medical technology consortium. ATI provided services that may closely support inherently governmental functions for the wearable diagnostics OTA, such as analyzing consortium members' cost proposals (see Figure 7).

---

[21] Office of Management and Budget, Office of Federal Procurement Policy, *Performance of Inherently Governmental and Critical Functions*, Policy Letter 11-01, 76 Fed. Reg. 56,227 (Sept. 12, 2011).

[22] The simplified acquisition threshold is generally $250,000. In certain situations, for domestic purchases, this threshold can be increased to $800,000. For example, the Office of Management and Budget noted that the President's emergency declaration related to COVID-19 allowed the simplified acquisition threshold to be increased. Currently, the simplified acquisition threshold for these purposes is $800,000.

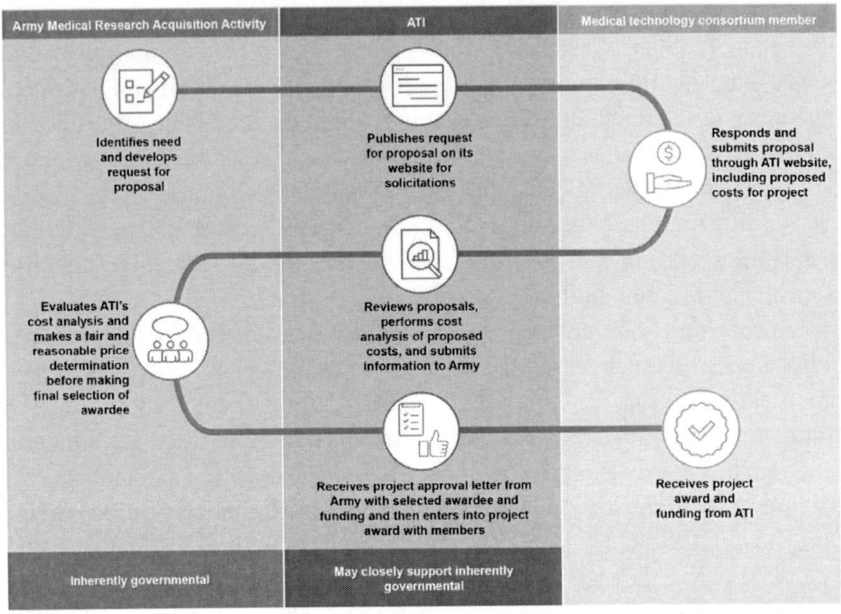

Source: GAO analysis of Army Medical Research Acquisition Activity and Advanced Technology International (ATI) information (data); iiierlok_xolms/stock.adobe.com (images). | GAO-21-501.

Figure 7. Examples of Services Performed by Advanced Technology International that May Closely Support Inherently Governmental Functions for a Coronavirus Disease 2019 Wearable Diagnostics Other Transaction Agreement.

The Army Medical Research Acquisition Activity agreements officer responsible for the wearable diagnostic devices OTA stated that, while ATI provided services that closely supported inherently governmental functions, the government ultimately retained control over its inherently governmental decisions. The agreements officer noted that he monitored ATI's performance to help ensure everyone "stayed in their lanes." For example, ATI conducted a cost analysis of the consortium members' cost proposals by reviewing proposed labor rates and comparing them to market rates, noting that the proposals provided sufficient cost data and were an adequate basis for award. The Army agreements officer then reviewed ATI's cost analysis and determined the costs to be fair and reasonable to the government. However, the agreements officer acknowledged that the Army Medical Research Acquisition Activity has limited contracting capacity, citing increased use of medical technology consortium OTA awards. ATI provides assistance in the government's evaluation process by providing cost analysis, which the agreements officer reviews, and administrative support. The agreements officer also confirmed that neither the base nor project OTA files included an assessment of the extent to which ATI was closely supporting inherently governmental functions or any enhanced management steps that needed to be planned for or taken to oversee ATI's performance of these activities. Since our review, Army officials plan to develop a process to measure and report on the consortium management's firm performance and a related quality assurance surveillance plan for the medical technology consortium OTA.

For the five OTAs that Army Contracting Command awarded through ATI to medical defense consortium members, Command officials also did not document an assessment of the extent to which ATI was closely supporting inherently governmental functions or any related enhanced management steps for overseeing ATI's performance in either the base or project OTAs. When we discussed this issue with an Army Contracting Command official in May 2021, the official told us that, upon review of the policy letter, it did not appear that ATI provides services that closely support inherently governmental functions. The official added that the agreement officers, agreement officer's representatives, and program officials responsible for these OTAs provide oversight of ATI's performance. A Command official also noted that the government's oversight responsibilities were reviewed and discussed during the acquisition planning phase, and that ATI performs services after receiving approval or authorization from an agreement officer or agreement officer's representative. Army Contracting Command has highlighted in its OTA training various acquisition support services provided by consortium management firms that could closely support inherently governmental functions, which are permitted. Specifically, typical consortium management duties include preparing requests for proposals; negotiating, awarding, and administering project OTAs; and project invoice receipt and payments. However, the training emphasized that the firms cannot perform inherently governmental functions. For the five medical defense consortium OTAs, ATI issued Army Contracting Command's request for proposals, entered into project OTAs on behalf of the government, and distributed funding to the OTA awardees. Without conducting and documenting an assessment of ATI's responsibilities, Army Contracting Command missed an opportunity to determine the extent to which ATI's services closely supported inherently governmental functions and to take any necessary steps to mitigate potential risks.

HHS's September 2012 and DOD's November 2018 OTA guides do not include information that agreements officers should consider when considering the use of a consortium management firm to support acquisition-related activities that could closely support inherently governmental functions.[23] The HHS OTA guide acknowledges that the roles and responsibilities of the participants in an OTA awarded through a consortium should be documented. However, the guide does not discuss the role of a consortium management firm specifically. HHS officials noted that they do not currently make much use of consortium management firms. However, as noted above, HHS officials stated they are interested in increasing use of consortiums in the future, which may lead to increased use of consortium management firms. Officials from DOD's Office of Defense Pricing and Contracting—the office responsible for updating DOD's OTA guide—noted that they are aware of risks associated with the functions provided by consortium management firms, such as performing services that closely support inherently governmental functions. Officials stated they are planning to update the DOD OTA guide to address such risks but did not offer time frames for when the update would be completed.

HHS's and DOD's guides also do not address what agreements officers should do after award to help ensure consortium management firms are not performing inherently governmental functions when they closely support such functions. For example, the guides do not direct agencies to monitor their oversight of consortium management firm activities to ensure they have sufficient capacity and capability to provide such oversight as needed. In contrast, DHS's July 2019 OTA guide states that agreements officers should, before and after award, ensure that consortium management firms are not performing inherently governmental functions.[24] The guide notes that the agreements officer should review the proposed scope of work of consortium management firms to identify functions that could be deemed inherently governmental and ensure that the OTA specified that the performance of such activities are conducted with sufficient federal involvement.

Without guidance on information that agreements officers should consider prior to awarding OTAs through consortia in which consortium management firms support acquisition-related activities, DOD and HHS agreements

---

[23] Department of Health and Human Services, Office of the Assistant Secretary for Preparedness and Response, Acquisition Management, Contracts and Grants, Biomedical Advanced Research and Development Authority, *Other Transaction Authority Guide and Standard Operating Procedure* (Sept. 2012) and Department of Defense, Office of the Under Secretary of Defense for Acquisition and Sustainment, *Other Transactions Guide, Version 1.0* (Nov. 2018).

[24] Department of Homeland Security, Office of the Chief Procurement Officer, *Other Transactions for Research and Prototype Projects Guide* (July 11, 2019).

officers may not fully consider the range of actions they should take to mitigate risks of consortium management firms if they perform functions that closely support inherently governmental functions.

DOD, HHS, and DHS Obligated $4.7 Billion on Undefinitized Contracts, but Contract Finalization Varied in Selected Cases

From March 2020 through March 2021, DOD, HHS, and DHS obligated $4.7 billion on undefinitized contracts in response to COVID-19 and definitized these contracts to varying degrees for the selected cases we reviewed. A majority of the $4.7 billion in contract obligations was for medical equipment and testing, hospital construction, drugs and biologicals, and support of the defense industrial base. DOD officials cited the ability to quickly award undefinitized contracts as a major benefit during COVID-19, while HHS and DHS used undefinitized contracts to a lesser extent.

Undefinitized Contracts Used to Acquire Medical Supplies and Services, Construct Hospitals, and Support Industrial Base

From March 2020 to March 2021, obligations on DOD, HHS, and DHS undefinitized contracts in response to COVID-19 increased from $250.3 million to about $4.7 billion. These undefinitized contract obligations comprised about 11 percent of COVID-19 procurement contract obligations across these three agencies as of March 14, 2021, with DOD accounting for the majority (see Table 4).

This 11 percent is slightly higher than in fiscal years 2017 through 2019, when obligations on DOD, HHS, and DHS's undefinitized contracts accounted for 8 to 10 percent of procurement contract obligations in each year.

Most of the COVID-19 obligations on undefinitized contracts awarded by DOD, HHS, and DHS were used to acquire medical equipment, testing, and drugs and biologicals; construct or alter hospitals; and support the defense industrial base (see Figure 8).

Table 4. DOD, HHS, and DHS undefinitized contract obligations in response to coronavirus disease 2019 as of March 14, 2021

Agency	**Undefinitized contract obligations ($)**	**Procurement contract obligations ($)**	**Undefinitized contract obligations as a percentage of procurement contract obligations (%)**
Department of Defense (DOD)	4 billion	24.1 billion	17
Department of Health and Human Services (HHS)	668 million	16 billion	4
Department of Homeland Security (DHS)	12 million	2.2 billion	1
Total	4.7 billion	42.2 billion	11

Source: GAO analysis of Federal Procurement Data System-Next Generation data. | GAO-21-501.

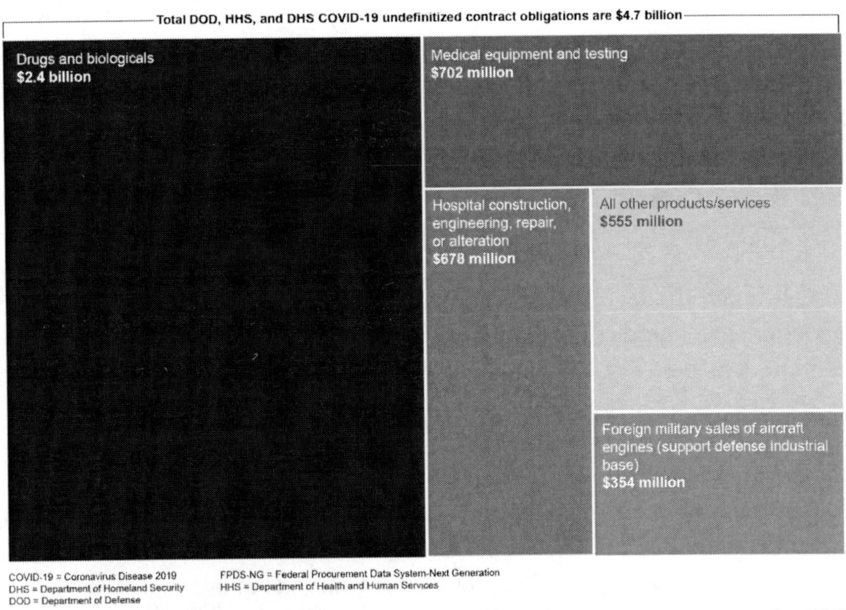

Note: Under the foreign military sales program, foreign governments pay the U.S. government to acquire defense articles and services on their behalf.

Source: GAO analysis of FPDS-NG data and information from DOD and HHS. | GAO-21-501.

Figure 8. Top COVID-19 Products and Services Acquired by DOD, HHS, and DHS Using Undefinitized Contracts as of March 14, 2021.

According to DOD officials, undefinitized contracts have been helpful in addressing COVID-19 because they allowed contractors to begin work immediately while they finalized negotiations. A senior DOD official stated that the ability to award an undefinitized contract on the same day that the agency receives funding is a powerful tool for responding to COVID-19. HHS officials stated that they did not make significant use of undefinitized contracts, in part, because many of their early purchases were for commercial products, which did not require undefinitized terms and conditions. DHS contracting policy officials stated that they did not make significant use of undefinitized contracts because they are not a preferred contracting mechanism within the department.

Following is additional information on the three undefinitized contracts we reviewed:

- *U.S. Army Corps of Engineers' undefinitized contract for an alternative care facility.* In March 2020, the Army Corps awarded a firm-fixed-price undefinitized contract with an estimated contract price of $101 million to Turner Construction, nearly 1 week after issuing the request for proposal. The contract was used to construct a temporary COVID-19 alternative care facility at Stony Brook University in New York.[25] According to a senior Army Corps official, the use of an undefinitized contract was imperative to building the facility as quickly as possible. When the Army Corps awarded the contract, terms and conditions such as the type, quantity, and location of equipment and structures had not yet been definitized.
  In May 2020, after the contract was definitized and the contractor completed construction of the facility, the State of New York took control of the facility. According to Army Corps officials, the facility was ready to be occupied when they turned it over to the State of New York. Army Corps officials emphasized that the State of New York did not require the facility to be permanent or designed to withstand adverse weather conditions. According to a senior Army Corps official, after construction completion, the facility experienced snow

[25] The facility was one of multiple facilities constructed throughout the U.S. by the Army Corps with disaster relief funding from the Federal Emergency Management Agency to help supplement the lack of capacity of existing hospitals. In April 2021, the DOD Inspector General reviewed the Army Corps' management of definitization timelines, fair and reasonable price determinations, and profits adjusted for costs incurred for 30 alternative care facility undefinitized contracts. For more information, see Department of Defense Inspector General, *Audit of the U.S. Army Corps of Engineers Use of Undefinitized Contract Actions for the Conversion of Alternate Care Sites in Response to the Coronavirus Disease–2019 Pandemic*, DODIG-2021-074 (Alexandria, VA: Apr. 7, 2021).

damage, wind damage, generator issues, and mold growth. The contractor maintained an on-site presence and worked with the Army Corps and the State of New York to resolve issues covered by the contractor's warranty during the 6-month warranty period. After the warranty period ended, the facility continued to experience weather-related damage and could no longer be occupied. The State of New York ultimately decided that the facility was not needed for patients, and the facility was never used. As of March 2021, the Army Corps obligated $155 million for this effort, which included an additional $54 million above the initial estimated price for items not included in the initial contract. These items included tents for putting on and taking off personal protective equipment.

- *ASPR undefinitized contract for convalescent plasma.* In March 2020, ASPR awarded a $750,000 undefinitized contract to the American Red Cross to start initial work for recruiting, collecting, and distributing convalescent plasma from individuals who have COVID-19 antibodies. ASPR awarded the undefinitized contract on the same day the program office received this requirement. ASPR officials stated that the undefinitized contract allowed the American Red Cross to begin work before officials had information on the delivery schedule or full scope of work. ASPR officials explained that none of the terms and conditions were definitized at the time of award because they did not have information on (1) the number of individuals who would be willing to donate plasma or (2) the start-up costs, such as marketing costs to recruit donors and the costs associated with the additional personal protective equipment needed to collect plasma from COVID- 19 patients. These officials also noted that the requirement was extraordinary and urgent because no other therapeutic options were available at the time.

  According to ASPR officials, when they definitized the contract in June 2020, the American Red Cross had already completed the necessary start-up work. According to ASPR officials, as of January 2021, the American Red Cross had collected over 142,000 units—at 200 milliliters per unit—of COVID-19 convalescent plasma and provided at least 1 unit of plasma to over 1,200 hospitals. As of March 2021, ASPR had obligated $120 million for this effort.
- *Air Force undefinitized contracts for aircraft engines.* In April 2020, the Air Force awarded four firm-fixed-price undefinitized contracts with a combined estimated total contract price of $707 million to

General Electric Aviation for foreign military sales of F110 engines to Slovakia, Bulgaria, Qatar, and Taiwan.[26] Prior to the COVID-19 pandemic, the Air Force had already planned to award undefinitized contracts for sales to Slovakia and Bulgaria because of the long-lead times for production.[27] COVID-19, however, caused a significant decrease in worldwide commercial airline travel, which created unprecedented challenges for aerospace companies reliant on commercial sales, including General Electric. As a result, General Electric requested that the Air Force also award undefinitized contracts for sales of engines to Qatar and Taiwan, as well as advance payments on all four undefinitized contracts.

The Air Force approved the requests, and according to Air Force officials, the only term not definitized at the time of award was the final negotiated price. Air Force officials explained that using undefinitized contracts for foreign military sales is a common practice because this allows the contractor to start work while the government works with the foreign nation on country-specific requirements. Similarly, we have previously found that DOD used undefinitized contracts for foreign military sales to help reduce schedule risk by allowing the work to start earlier than under a definitized contract.[28]

Timing of Definitization and Amount Obligated Prior to Definitization

Table 5 shows the timing of definitization and the amounts obligated for the three undefinitized contracts we reviewed.

---

[26] The foreign military sales program is an acquisition process through which the U.S. government procures military equipment, training, and other services on behalf of foreign governments. The Arms Export Control Act authorizes the sale of defense articles and services to eligible foreign customers under this program, which is one of multiple security cooperation programs that provide for the transfer of defense articles and services to foreign governments.

[27] Long-lead items include aircraft engines, which need to be procured early to reduce production lead times and ensure that planned production schedules are maintained for the related end item—the aircraft.

[28] GAO, *Foreign Military Sales: Expanding Use of Tools to Sufficiently Define Requirements Could Enable More Timely Acquisitions,* GAO-17-682 (Washington, D.C.: Aug. 14, 2017).

Table 5. Definitization timing and amounts obligated for selected undefinitized contracts awarded in response to coronavirus disease 2019 (COVID-19)

Description of undefinitized contract and the contracting agency	Time between award and definitization	Amount obligated prior to definitization
Alternative care facility in Stony Brook, New York (U.S. Army Corps of Engineers)	22 days	$101 million or 100 percent of the estimated contract price[a]
COVID-19 convalescent plasma (Department of Health and Human Services, Office of the Assistant Secretary for Preparedness and Response)	72 days	$750,000 or 100 percent of the initial estimated contract price[b]
Foreign military sales of F110 engines to support defense industrial base (Air Force)[c]	Not applicable – not yet definitized as of April 12, 2021, 349 days after award	$354 million or 50 percent of the estimated contract price

Source: GAO analysis of Department of Defense and Department of Health and Human Services information. | GAO-21-501.

[a]The CARES Act grants additional flexibilities for DOD to waive certain limitations on the amounts that can be obligated before the contract is definitized.

[b]The initial estimated contract price of $750,000, obligated at the time of award, was ultimately less than 1 percent of the total obligated amount on the undefinitized contract as of March 14, 2021 ($120 million).

[c]The Air Force took actions to increase cash flow to the contractor to offset financial distress caused by COVID-19.

Agency officials provided additional context for the obligation amounts and timing of definitization for these three undefinitized contracts:

- Pursuant to the CARES Act, the Army Corps' head of contracting activity approved a class waiver that removed certain statutory and regulatory limitations on obligations for all alternative care facility undefinitized contracts, including the Stony Brook contract.[29] Specifically, the waiver permitted Army Corps contracting personnel to obligate 100 percent of the estimated contract price prior to definitization. According to the determination, the Army Corps was the only entity with the capacity to build the temporary medical infrastructure needed to support rapid response to COVID-19. The determination further noted that definitizing the undefinitized contract at 50 percent of the estimated contract price (or 75 percent

[29] Pub. L. No. 116-136, § 13005, 134 Stat. at 522.

with a qualifying proposal from the contractor) would have risked unacceptable construction delay for this significant and high priority mission.

- For the COVID-19 convalescent plasma undefinitized contract, ASPR officials explained that they determined the initial estimated contract price to be $750,000 and obligated this full amount at award. As noted earlier, ASPR officials did not have information related to the price per unit, quantities, or start-up costs. As a result, they did not include a total estimated contract price in their justification for using an undefinitized contract, which is inconsistent with HHS's acquisition procedures.[30] ASPR officials explained that given the urgency of the requirement and lack of information, including an estimated cost for the total effort was not feasible at the time. According to ASPR officials, the senior officials responsible for approving the undefinitized contract knew that the total effort would be greater than the initial $750,000 and that the risks of starting the undefinitized contract without key information far outweighed risks of waiting for more information given the lives being lost to COVID-19. ASPR officials definitized the contract after obligating the initial $750,000, which accounted for less than 1 percent of the $120 million obligated on the contract as of March 14, 2021.
- For the four foreign military sales undefinitized contracts, Air Force officials stated that they had not yet definitized the contracts 349 days after award because General Electric had not yet submitted a qualifying proposal. DOD may only enter into an undefinitized contract if it requires definitization of contractual terms, specifications, and price within 180 days after the contractor submits a qualifying proposal for definitization or before obligating 50 percent of the estimated contract price, whichever occurs earlier.[31] The CARES Act allowed DOD to waive these requirements. However, the Air Force has not elected to waive these requirements for the four foreign military sales undefinitized contracts.[32]

[30] Department of Health and Human Services; Health and Human Services Acquisition Regulation; Policy, Guidance, and Instructions § 316.603-70.
[31] 10 U.S.C. § 2326(b).
[32] Pub. L. No. 116-136, § 13005, 134 Stat. at 522.

Conclusion

Federal contracting—including OTAs—plays a critical role in the nation's response to COVID-19 by accelerating the development of vaccines and the procurement of vital goods and services. It is imperative for the public and congressional decision makers to understand the significant role that OTAs play and how they can be leveraged in the future, especially if another national emergency calls for the expanded use of such tools. Government-wide systems can improve OTA reporting, but only if agencies collectively prioritize and implement these changes. Further, it is also critical that agencies provide greater insight and oversight on consortium management firms that may perform functions that are closely associated with inherently governmental functions. This will contribute to greater transparency and help ensure that the firms do not perform inherently governmental functions.

Recommendations for Executive Action

We are making a total of 14 recommendations, including four to DOD, four to DHS, two to GSA, and four to HHS. Specifically:

The Secretary of Defense—in coordination with the change control board governing the Integrated Award Environment—should consider prioritizing the development and implementation of a systematic approach to consistently and accurately track other transaction agreements used for national interest events and the associated dollars obligated. (Recommendation 1)

The Secretary of Homeland Security—in coordination with the change control board governing the Integrated Award Environment—should consider prioritizing the development and implementation of a systematic approach to consistently and accurately track other transaction agreements used for national interest events and the associated dollars obligated. (Recommendation 2)

The Secretary of Health and Human Services—in coordination with the change control board governing the Integrated Award Environment— should consider prioritizing the development and implementation of a systematic approach to consistently and accurately track other transaction agreements used for national interest events and the associated dollars obligated. (Recommendation 3)

The Administrator of the General Services Administration—in coordination with the change control board governing the Integrated Award

Environment—should consider prioritizing the development and implementation of a systematic approach to consistently and accurately track other transaction agreements used for national interest events and the associated dollars obligated. (Recommendation 4)

Until a systematic approach to consistently and accurately track other transaction agreements used for national interest events is implemented, the Secretary of Homeland Security should update Department of Homeland Security guidance to clarify how other transaction agreements awarded in response to COVID-19 should be designated when reporting in the other transaction agreement module of the Federal Procurement Data System-Next Generation. (Recommendation 5)

The Secretary of Defense—in coordination with the change control board governing the Integrated Award Environment—should consider prioritizing the development and implementation of a systematic approach to track the consortium members performing for each other transaction agreement awarded through a consortium or consortium management firm. (Recommendation 6)

The Secretary of Homeland Security—in coordination with the change control board governing the Integrated Award Environment—should consider prioritizing the development and implementation of a systematic approach to track the consortium members performing for each other transaction agreement awarded through a consortium or consortium management firm. (Recommendation 7)

The Secretary of Health and Human Services—in coordination with the change control board governing the Integrated Award Environment— should consider prioritizing the development and implementation of a systematic approach to track the consortium members performing for each other transaction agreement awarded through a consortium or consortium management firm. (Recommendation 8)

The Administrator of the General Services Administration—in coordination with the change control board governing the Integrated Award Environment—should consider prioritizing the development and implementation of a systematic approach to track the consortium members performing for each other transaction agreement awarded through a consortium or consortium management firm. (Recommendation 9)

Until a systematic approach to track consortium members for other transaction agreements awarded through a consortium or consortium management firm is implemented, the Secretary of Defense should provide information to the public and congressional decision makers on the consortium members performing on each other transaction agreement awarded through a consortium or consortium management firm, such as by including this information in the description of requirement field in the other transaction agreement module of the Federal Procurement Data System-Next Generation. (Recommendation 10)

Until a systematic approach to track consortium members for other transaction agreements awarded through a consortium or consortium management firm is implemented, the Secretary of Health and Human Services should direct the Office of the Assistant Secretary for Preparedness and Response to provide information to the public and congressional decision makers on the consortium members performing on each other transaction agreement awarded through a consortium or consortium management firm, such as by including this information in the description of requirement field in the other transaction agreement module of the Federal Procurement Data System-Next Generation. (Recommendation 11)

Until a systematic approach to track consortium members for other transaction agreements awarded through a consortium or consortium management firm is implemented across agencies, the Secretary of Homeland Security should provide information to the public on the consortium members performing on each other transaction agreement awarded through a consortium or consortium management firm, such as by including this information in the description of requirement field in the other transaction agreement module of Federal Procurement Data System-Next Generation. (Recommendation 12)

The Secretary of Defense should direct the Director of Defense Pricing and Contracting to update the Department of Defense's other transaction agreement guidance to include what agreement officers should consider when planning to use a consortium management firm to support acquisition-related activities, such as assessing the extent to which a consortium management firm is closely supporting inherently governmental functions and, for firms that do so, what enhanced management oversight activities are appropriate, if any. (Recommendation 13)

The Secretary of Health and Human Services should direct the Assistant Secretary for Preparedness and Response to update the Department of Health and Human Services' other transaction agreement guidance to include what agreement officers should consider when planning to use a consortium management firm to support acquisition-related activities, such as assessing the extent to which a consortium management firm is closely supporting inherently governmental functions and, for firms that do so, what enhanced management oversight activities are appropriate, if any. (Recommendation 14)

Agency Comments and Our Evaluation

We provided a draft of this report to DOD, HHS, DHS, and GSA for review and comment. In written comments provided by DOD, HHS, DHS, and GSA (reproduced in appendices II, III, IV, and V), the agencies concurred with 11 of the 14 recommendations. Specifically, DOD concurred with three of four recommendations, HHS concurred with all four, DHS concurred with two of four, and GSA concurred with both recommendations. The agencies generally provided steps they plan to take to address these recommendations. As discussed further below, DOD partially concurred with one recommendation, and DHS did not concur with two recommendations—all three related to consistently and accurately tracking OTAs awarded in response to national interest events and dollars obligated.

DOD concurred with recommendations 6, 10, and 13 and described its plans to address these recommendations in its written comments. DOD partially concurred with the first recommendation regarding consideration to prioritize the development and implementation of a systematic approach to consistently and accurately track OTAs used for national interest events and the associated dollars obligated. In its written comments, DOD noted that it understands the importance of being able to quickly identify awards made in support of national emergencies, such as the response to the COVID-19 pandemic, for the public. DOD further notes that the federal response to COVID-19 is very unique, and it is unlikely that OTAs will be used to respond to national emergencies, natural disasters, or contingency actions in the future. As a result, DOD stated it does not believe expending resources on system changes to FPDS-NG is warranted.

However, as we noted in our report, prior to the start of the pandemic, DOD, DHS, and HHS increased their use of OTAs from $2.4 billion in fiscal year 2017 to $7.8 billion in fiscal year 2019, or a 225 percent increase. Further, in response to COVID-19, agencies obligated about $12 billion on OTAs for research, development, and manufacturing purposes. As future national emergencies arise—whether they are natural disasters, contingency operations, or another health crisis—OTAs will likely play a role in such events.

Through the Integrated Award Environment's change control board, agencies have an opportunity to lay the groundwork for better transparency on OTA awards for national interest events in the future. In its written comments, DOD also noted that a process-based approach, rather than FPDS-NG system changes, could help track such OTAs, and that it would work with the Integrated Award Environment's change control board to consider different approaches for identifying OTA awards in the future. As the recommendation did not specify that the systematic tracking should be accomplished through FPDS-NG changes, we believe that DOD's planned actions could meet the intent of the recommendation.

HHS concurred with recommendations 3, 8, 11, and 14 and described its plans to address these recommendations in its written comments. In its response, HHS shared plans to work in coordination with DOD and DHS to prioritize the development of a systematic approach to consistently and accurately track OTAs used for national interest events and to track the consortium members performing for each OTA awarded through a consortium or consortium management firm.

DHS concurred with recommendations 7 and 12 and described its plans to address these recommendations in its written comments. DHS did not concur with the second recommendation regarding consideration to prioritize the development and implementation of a systematic approach to consistently and accurately track OTAs used for national interest events and the associated dollars obligated. In its written comments, DHS noted that only its research and prototype OTAs are required by statute to be reported in FPDS-NG. However, the primary purpose of the recommendation is to increase accuracy and transparency for the public to better understand the use of OTAs and dollars obligated, regardless of what is required by statute to be publicly reported. Regardless of what OTAs are required to be reported, DHS reported its use of OTAs to FPDS-NG, and the reporting was inaccurate. As we noted in our report, DHS obligated $57 million on COVID-19 OTAs, and of that, $25.5 million or about 45 percent had not been accurately identified by DHS as COVID-19-related. Further, none of the $57 million on DHS's COVID-19 OTAs were research and prototype OTAs. Instead, all of DHS's COVID- 19 OTAs were awarded by either the Countering Weapons of Mass Destruction Office or Transportation Security Administration for services, such as airport screening and cleaning. The discrepancy between what DHS is statutorily required to report and what it actually reports for OTAs underscores the inconsistency of reporting within DHS and the need for quality information about OTA use and dollars in response to national interest events.

In its response, DHS stated that if there is future use of OTAs in response to a national interest event, DHS will issue instructions on how to identify those actions when reporting to FPDS-NG is required. We believe there are shortcomings to such an approach. The lack of a systematic approach is, in part, why there was inaccurate reporting of COVID-19 OTAs. While it is not possible to anticipate the types of national interest events that may arise in the future, DHS has an opportunity to approach OTA reporting in a proactive rather than reactive manner.

DHS's response also noted that FPDS-NG is used for reporting summary level details of awards rather than dollars. However, this is an inaccurate portrayal of FPDS-NG. FPDS-NG is the authoritative source for contracting data, which includes dollars obligated on contract actions, and is used by federal agencies to create reports to the President, the Congress, GAO, federal agencies, and the public. As we noted in our report, DHS obligated $57 million on OTAs in response to COVID-19 based on FPDS-NG data. In addition, FPDS-NG is a public database that provides insight into summary-level OTA spending (agencies have not reported data on OTAs in USAspending.gov). The recommendation is meant to start a dialogue among the Integrated Award Environment's change control board agencies to weigh the costs and benefits of a systematic approach to allow accurate and consistent tracking of OTA obligations for decision makers and the public.

While DHS requests the recommendation be resolved and closed, given the reasons that we cited above, we continue to believe that DHS should consider prioritizing the development and implementation of a systematic approach to accurately and consistently track OTAs used for national interest events and the associated dollars obligated.

DHS also did not concur with the fifth recommendation regarding updating DHS guidance to clarify how OTAs awarded in response to COVID-19 should be designated when reporting in the OTA module of FPDS-NG. In its response, DHS noted that additional guidance is not necessary because designation of OTAs is addressed in its July 2019 OTA guide, and that only research and prototype OTAs are required to be reported in FPDS-NG. However, DHS's response does not address the primary purpose of the recommendation—to provide the public with better transparency on the dollars obligated on COVID-19 OTAs. First, DHS's July 2019 OTA guide pre-dates COVID-19 and thus does not address how DHS should identify COVID-19 OTAs. Further, as noted above, regardless of what DHS is required to report in FPDS-NG, it did not accurately identify 45 percent of reported OTA dollars as COVID-19- related.

DHS's response noted that DHS voluntarily entered all of its Countering Weapons of Mass Destruction OTAs into FPDS-NG in response to COVID-19. However, without guidance to contracting personnel, it is likely that there will continue to be errors in reporting. As we noted in our report, part of the reason why DHS did not accurately identify $25.5 million in OTAs as COVID-19-related is because DHS lacks guidance instructing contracting personnel to do so. In its response, DHS also noted that it maintains an internal OTA data collection and tracking log to ensure OTAs are being documented. While this may be a helpful agency management tool, such information is not publicly available and does not provide the public with transparency into DHS's COVID-19 OTAs.

While DHS requests the recommendation be resolved and closed, given the reasons that we cited above, we continue to believe that DHS should update DHS guidance to clarify how OTAs awarded in response to COVID-19 should be designated when reporting in the OTA module of FPDS-NG.

GSA concurred with recommendations 4 and 9 and described its plans to address these recommendations in its written comments. In its response, GSA recognized that policy drives the Integrated Award Environment system functionality and noted it will collaborate with executive branch stakeholders to clarify existing policy guidance on agency reporting requirements for OTAs. GSA also noted it will work with the Integrated Award Environment's change control board to identify opportunities to enhance OTA tracking and reporting compliance.

DOD, HHS, and DHS also provided technical comments, which we incorporated as appropriate.

We are sending copies of this report to the appropriate congressional committees, the Administrator of the General Services Administration, the Secretary of Defense, the Secretary of Health and Human Services, the Secretary of Homeland Security, and other interested parties. In addition, the report is available at no charge on the GAO website at http://www.gao.gov.

If you or your staff have any questions about this report, please contact me at (202) 512-4841 or makm@gao.gov. Contact points for our Offices of Congressional Relations and Public Affairs may be found on the last page of this report. GAO staff who made key contributions to the report are listed in appendix VI.

Marie A. Mak; Director, Contracting and National Security Acquisitions

List of Committees

The Honorable Patrick Leahy
Chairman
The Honorable Richard Shelby
Vice Chairman
Committee on Appropriations
United States Senate

The Honorable Ron Wyden
Chairman
The Honorable Mike Crapo
Ranking Member Committee on Finance
United States Senate

The Honorable Patty Murray
Chair
The Honorable Richard Burr
Ranking Member
Committee on Health, Education, Labor, and Pensions
United States Senate

The Honorable Gary C. Peters
Chairman
The Honorable Rob Portman
Ranking Member
Committee on Homeland Security and Governmental Affairs
United States Senate

The Honorable Rosa L. DeLauro
Chairwoman
The Honorable Kay Granger
Ranking Member
Committee on Appropriations
House of Representatives

The Honorable Frank Pallone, Jr.
Chairman
The Honorable Cathy McMorris Rodgers
Republican Leader
Committee on Energy and Commerce
House of Representatives

The Honorable Bennie G. Thompson
Chairman
The Honorable John Katko
Ranking Member
Committee on Homeland Security
House of Representatives

The Honorable Carolyn B. Maloney
Chairwoman
The Honorable James Comer
Ranking Member
Committee on Oversight and Reform
House of Representatives

The Honorable Richard E. Neal
Chairman
The Honorable Kevin Brady
Republican Leader
Committee on Ways and Means
House of Representatives

Appendix I: Objectives, Scope, and Methodology

This report examines the extent to which: (1) selected agencies used other transaction agreements (OTA) in response to Coronavirus Disease 2019 (COVID-19), and what factors contributed to their use, (2) these COVID-19 OTAs were awarded to consortia and how agencies provided oversight, and (3) selected agencies used and managed undefinitized contracts in response to COVID-19.

To identify the extent to which selected agencies used OTAs in response to COVID-19, we identified all the agencies that reported obligating dollars through OTAs in response to COVID-19 in the Federal Procurement Database System-Next Generation (FPDS-NG).[1] These agencies were:

- Department of Defense (DOD);[2]
- Department of Health and Human Services (HHS)—specifically, the Office of the Assistant Secretary for Preparedness and Response (ASPR), which includes the Biomedical Advanced Research and Development Authority;[3] and
- Department of Homeland Security (DHS)—specifically, the Countering Weapons of Mass Destruction Office and the Transportation Security Administration.

We analyzed data available in the OTA module of FPDS-NG as of March 14, 2021 and identified OTAs and associated obligations by searching for "coronavirus" and "COVID-19" in the description of requirement data field. We analyzed the FPDS-NG data to identify the types of goods or services procured by DOD, HHS, and DHS using OTAs. We assessed the reliability of the FPDS-NG data by reviewing existing information about the FPDS-NG system and the data it collects, such as the data dictionary and data validation rules; performing electronic testing; and comparing reported data to agency-

---

[1] FPDS-NG is a comprehensive, web-based tool for agencies to report procurement contract actions and is the authoritative source for procurement award data, including dollars obligated on contract actions. It also includes a module for reporting OTAs.

[2] While DOD can use OTAs for research, prototyping, and production purposes, this report is focused only on OTAs used to support prototyping and production efforts.

[3] The National Institutes of Health—a part of HHS—did not report awarding any OTAs in response to COVID-19 in FPDS-NG as of March 14, 2021. In May 2021, officials from the National Institutes of Health informed us they had obligated about $520 million on COVID-19 OTAs as of April 26, 2021. We did not assess the reliability of these data and did not include the $520 million in our analysis.

provided data and OTA documents. We determined that the control activities component of internal controls was significant to this objective, along with the principle that management should design information systems and related control activities to achieve objectives and respond to risks. We also determined that the information and communication component of internal controls was significant to this objective, along with the principle that management should externally communicate quality information to achieve objectives. We assessed the FPDS-NG OTA module system and its ability to accurately provide quality data on the actions and associated obligations for COVID-19 OTAs and the extent to which this information was communicated to congressional decision makers and the public. We found the agencies did not accurately report all COVID-19 OTA obligations, which we further discuss in the report. We identified additional COVID-19 OTA obligations through agency-provided data and documents. After we corrected the FPDS-NG OTA data for the inaccuracies and underreporting, we determined the data were sufficiently reliable for the purposes of describing agencies' reported OTA obligations in response to COVID-19. We also interviewed officials from the General Services Administration (GSA), which administers FPDS-NG, including the OTA module.

To identify the factors that contributed to DOD, HHS, and DHS using OTAs in selected cases, we selected a nongeneralizable sample of 15 OTAs awarded between February 2020 and October 2020 based on the FPDS-NG data, using the following criteria:[4]

- Highest dollars obligated
- Representation of all three contracting agencies
- Mix of product or service acquired
- Vendor, including consortium participation
- Justification for OTA use (nontraditional contractor participation, cost sharing, exceptional circumstance)
- Type of OTA (prototype or production)
- OTAs with potential data reliability concerns, including those identified by agencies as COVID-19-related but were not identified as COVID- 19 in FPDS-NG

[4] Our selected OTAs included those awarded prior to February 2020 but were modified between February 2020 and October 2020 to include COVID-19 work.

Table 6. Selected COVID-19 Other Transaction Agreements (OTA)

Agency/component - vendor (consortium participation)	**OTA number**	**Description**	**Obligations as of March 14, 2021 ($)**
HHS/ASPR - Janssen (not through a consortium)	HHSO100201700018C	COVID-19 vaccine development and clinical studies	1.1 billion
DOD/Army Contracting Command - Janssen (through a consortium)	W15QKN1691002 P000081	COVID-19 vaccine manufacturing	1 billion
HHS/ASPR - AstraZeneca (not through a consortium)	75A50120C00114	COVID-19 vaccine development	126 million
DOD/Army Contracting Command - AstraZeneca (not through a consortium)	W15QKN2191003	COVID-19 vaccine development and manufacturing	1.2 billion
DOD/Army Contracting Command - Sanofi (through a consortium)	W15QKN1691002 P000078	COVID-19 vaccine manufacturing	1.8 billion
DOD/Army Contracting Command - Novavax (through a consortium)	W15QKN1691002 P000074[a]	COVID-19 vaccine manufacturing	1.6 billion
DOD/Army Contracting Command - Pfizer (through a consortium)	W15QKN1691002 P000076	COVID-19 vaccine manufacturing	2 billion
DOD/Army Contracting Command - Cue Inc. (not through a consortium)	W911NF2190001	Nonvaccine: increase domestic production capacity of COVID-19 rapid detection test kits	481 million
DOD/Army Medical Research Acquisition Activity – University of California, San Francisco/Empatica/Sempulse/Fitbit/Diomics/Silbel/ Philips (through a consortium)	W81XWH2090015	Nonvaccine: the development of wearable diagnostics for COVID-19 detection	19.2 million
DHS/Countering Weapons of Mass Destruction - American Medical Response (not through a consortium)	70RWMD20T00000006	Nonvaccine: COVID-19 screening at U.S. Customs and Border Protection federal inspection stations within ports of entry	23 million

DHS/Transportation Security Administration - City of Atlanta, Department of Aviation (not through a consortium)	HSTS0116HRES950	Nonvaccine: COVID-19 cleaning and sanitation at the Atlanta Airport	4.9 million
DOD/Air Force - Essentium Inc. (not through a consortium)	FA86492099135	Nonvaccine: 3D printing for replacement parts to support the industrial base[b]	4.25 million
DOD/Army Contracting Command - Augustine Consulting, Inc. (not through a consortium)	W91CRB2090001	Nonvaccine: crisis response communication kit	11 million
HHS/ASPR - Regeneron Pharmaceuticals (not through a consortium)	HHSO100201700020C	Nonvaccine: COVID-19 therapeutic development	231 million
DOD/Army Contracting Command - Regeneron Pharmaceuticals, Inc. (through a consortium)	W15QKN1691002 P00074[a]	Nonvaccine: large scale manufacturing of COVID-19 therapeutic	450 million

ASPR - Office of the Assistant Secretary for Preparedness and Response

COVID-19 - Coronavirus Disease 2019

DHS - Department of Homeland Security DOD - Department of Defense

HHS - Department of Health and Human Services

Source: GAO review of Federal Procurement Data System-Next Generation and agency information. | GAO-21-501

[a]The OTA modification included two awards—one to Novavax and one to Regeneron.

[b]The Air Force took actions to increase cash flow to the contractor to offset financial distress caused by COVID-19.

When we selected our sample of OTAs in October 2020, the obligations on OTAs across DOD, HHS, and DHS were 30 percent of total obligations on all contracting mechanisms—OTAs and procurement contracts—for these three agencies.

We selected seven vaccine OTAs, which comprised all obligations on COVID-19 vaccine OTAs. We also selected eight nonvaccine OTAs. See Table 6 for details on the OTAs we selected.

The seven selected vaccine OTAs awarded by DOD and HHS account for all $8.9 billion obligated on COVID-19 vaccine OTAs. The selected eight nonvaccine OTAs awarded by DOD, HHS, and DHS accounted for an additional $1.2 billion in COVID-19 obligations. Combined, these 15 OTAs accounts for 81 percent of all obligation on COVID-19 OTAs as of March 14, 2021. For these selected cases, we analyzed OTA documents, such as written determinations for OTA use, solicitation documents, and award documents, and interviewed agreements officers and program officials. As part of our analysis, we determined the extent to which these OTAs used available CARES Act flexibilities. In addition, we reviewed agencies' OTA policies and guidance and interviewed contracting policy officials at DOD, HHS, and DHS.

To identify the extent to which DOD, HHS, and DHS awarded OTAs to consortia in response to COVID-19, we analyzed the same data available in the OTA module of FPDS-NG as discussed above but by vendor, and we supplemented this analysis with reviews of publicly available information and OTA documents. We determined that the information and communication component of internal controls was significant to this objective, along with the principle that management should externally communicate quality information to achieve objectives. We assessed DOD's, HHS's, and DHS's efforts to provide quality data on the consortium members who performed significant work on OTAs to congressional decision makers and the public. Of the 15 selected OTA cases we reviewed, six were awarded to consortia, all by DOD. To determine how DOD provided oversight for these six OTAs, we analyzed OTA documents and interviewed agreements officers and program officials to identify the extent to which these OTAs included analysis required by the Office of Federal Procurement Policy's Policy Letter 11-01 when contractors perform work closely associated with inherently governmental functions.[1] We reviewed DOD, HHS, and DHS policies related to OTAs

[1] Office of Management and Budget, Office of Federal Procurement Policy, *Performance of Inherently Governmental and Critical Functions*, Policy Letter 11-01, 76 Fed. Reg. 56,227 (Sept. 12, 2011).

awarded to consortia and these agencies' reports to congressional committees regarding OTA use. We also interviewed officials from Advanced Technology International (ATI), the consortium management firm that received the majority of COVID-19 OTA obligations according to FPDS-NG data.

To identify the extent to which DOD, HHS, and DHS used undefinitized contracts in response to COVID-19, we analyzed data available in the procurement contract module of FPDS-NG as of March 14, 2021.[2] We primarily identified these contract actions and associated obligations related to the COVID-19 response by using the National Interest Action code and supplementing this analysis by searching for "coronavirus" and "COVID-19" in the description of requirement data field.[3] For the purposes of our analysis, undefinitized contract obligations are associated with contract actions identified in FPDS-NG as undefinitized, which includes letter contracts. DOD, HHS, and DHS accounted for 96 percent of all COVID-19-related undefinitized contract obligations reported across the federal government in FPDS-NG over the time frame of our review, or $4.9 billion. We analyzed the FPDS-NG data to identify the types of goods or services procured by DOD, HHS, and DHS using undefinitized contracts. We assessed the reliability of the FPDS-NG data by reviewing existing information about the FPDS-NG system and the data it collects, such as the data dictionary and data validation rules; performing electronic testing, and comparing reported data to source documents. We determined the FPDS-NG data were sufficiently reliable for the purposes of describing agencies' reported undefinitized contract obligations in response to COVID-19.

To identify how DOD, HHS, and DHS managed selected undefinitized contracts, we selected a nongeneralizable sample of three undefinitized contracts awarded between February 2020 and October 2020 based on the FPDS-NG data, using the following criteria:

---

[2] On April 12, 2021, in response to our review, HHS corrected information for an undefinitized contract we reviewed by revising nine actions from being incorrectly identified as undefinitized to correctly identified as definitized. We incorporated these revisions into our March 14, 2021 data analysis, which resulted in a reduction of HHS undefinitized contract obligations by $120 million.

[3] National Interest Action codes were established in 2005 after Hurricane Katrina with the purpose of tracking federal procurements for specific disasters, emergencies, or contingency events.

- Highest dollars obligated
- Representation of the contracting agencies with the majority of undefinitized contract obligations (DOD and HHS)
- Mix of product or service acquired
- Definitization status and schedule
- Percentage of work completed before definitization
- Vendor
- Extent competed

When we selected our sample of undefinitized contracts, the obligations on undefinitized contracts across the three agencies were 6 percent of total obligations on all contracting mechanisms—OTAs and procurement contracts.

See Table 7 for details on the undefinitized contracts we selected.

The three undefinitized contracts we selected were awarded by DOD and HHS and had combined undefinitized contract obligations of $509 million or about 10 percent of all COVID-19 undefinitized contract obligations. For these selected cases, we analyzed contract documents, such as written determinations and award documents, and interviewed contracting officers and program officials. As part of our analysis, we determined the extent to which DOD used available CARES Act flexibilities for its undefinitized contracts. In addition, we reviewed the Federal Acquisition Regulation, agencies' federal acquisition regulation supplements, and agency policies and guidance related to undefinitized contracts. We also interviewed contracting policy officials at DOD, HHS, and DHS.

We conducted this performance audit from August 2020 to July 2021 in accordance with generally accepted government auditing standards. Those standards require that we plan and perform the audit to obtain sufficient, appropriate evidence to provide a reasonable basis for our findings and conclusions based on our audit objectives. We believe that the evidence obtained provides a reasonable basis for our findings and conclusions based on our audit objectives.

Table 7. Selected COVID-19 undefinitized contracts

Agency/component - vendor	**Contract number**	**Description**	**Obligations as of March 14, 2021 ($)**
DOD/Air Force - General Electric Company	FA862618D0029 (base award), FA862620F0026 (delivery order), FA862620F0027 (delivery order), FA862620F0028 (delivery order), FA862620F0029 (delivery order)	Foreign military sales of jet engines to four countries to support the defense industrial base[a]	353.6 million
DOD/Army Corps of Engineers - Turner Construction Company	W912DS20C0008	Construct an alternative care facility in Stony Brook, New York	154.6 million
HHS/ASPR - American Red Cross	75A50120C00045	Convalescent plasma coordination and distribution	120.3 million[b]

ASPR - Office of the Assistant Secretary for Preparedness and Response

COVID-19 - Coronavirus Disease 2019

DOD - Department of Defense

HHS - Department of Health and Human Services

Source: GAO review of Federal Procurement Data System-Next Generation and agency information. | GAO-21-501.

[a]The Air Force took actions to increase cash flow to the contractor to offset financial distress caused by COVID-19.

[b]Of the $120.3 million in obligations, HHS obligated $750,000 prior to definitizing or finalizing the contract and $119.6 million after definitizing the contract.

Appendix II: Comments from the Department of Defense

OFFICE OF THE UNDER SECRETARY OF DEFENSE
3000 DEFENSE PENTAGON
WASHINGTON, DC 20301-3000

ACQUISITION
AND SUSTAINMENT

Ms. Marie Mak
Director, Contracting and National Security
U.S. Government Accountability Office
441 G Street, NW
Washington DC 20548

Dear Ms. Mak,

This is the Department of Defense response to GAO Draft Report GAO-21-501, "COVID-19 CONTRACTING: Actions Needed to Enhance Transparency and Oversight of Selected Awards," dated June 4, 2021 (GAO Code 104497).

Enclosed is the Department's response to the subject report. My point of contact is Mr. Gregory Snyder who can be reached at gregory.d.snyder.civ@mail.mil and or 703-614-0719.

Sincerely,

TENAGLIA.JOHN.M.1154945926 Digitally signed by TENAGLIA.JOHN.M.1154945926 Date: 2021.07.09 10:50:34 -04'00'

John M. Tenaglia
Principal Director,
Defense Pricing and Contracting

Enclosure:
As stated

Enclosure

GAO DRAFT REPORT DATED JUNE 4, 2021
GAO-21-501 (GAO CODE 104497)

"COVID-19 CONTRACTING: ACTIONS NEEDED TO ENHANCE TRANSPARENCY AND OVERSIGHT OF SELECTED AWARDS"

DEPARTMENT OF DEFENSE COMMENTS TO THE GAO RECOMMENDATION

DoD RECOMMENDATION 1: The Secretary of Defense—in coordination with the change control board governing the Integrated Award Environment—should consider prioritizing the development and implementation of a systematic approach to consistently and accurately track Other Transaction Authorities (OTAs) used for national interest events and the associated dollars obligated. (Recommendation 1)

DoD RESPONSE: Partially Concur. The Department understands the importance of being able to quickly identify awards made in support of national emergencies, such as the response to the COVID-19 pandemic, for the public. However, in addition to an approach that would change the Federal Procurement Data System (FPDS) as recommended, DoD believes there are process-based approaches that could satisfy the need for identifying related Other Transactions for Prototypes / Production awards that would not require additional resources at FPDS or the agency-level to implement. Notwithstanding the very unique COVID-19 pandemic federal response, it is unlikely that Other Transactions for Prototypes / Production would routinely be used in the future to respond to other National Emergencies, natural disasters, or contingency actions; and, as such, expending resources on system changes to FPDS and agency contract writing systems may not be warranted. Regardless, DoD will work with the agency members of the change control board as necessary to consider different approaches and develop a standard framework for how agencies can identify applicable Other Transactions for Prototype / Production awards in the future.

DoD RECOMMENDATION 2: The Secretary of Defense—in coordination with the change control board governing the Integrated Award Environment—should consider prioritizing the development and implementation of a systematic approach to track the consortium members performing for each OTA awarded through a consortium or consortium management firm. (Recommendation 6)

DoD RESPONSE: Concur. The Department recognizes the need to more easily identify the individual consortium member performing on an order awarded to the consortium. DoD will work with the federal change control board to propose a method for doing so as part of reporting OTs for Prototypes/Production to the FPDS.

DoD RECOMMENDATION 3: Until a systematic approach to track consortium members for OTAs awarded through a consortium or consortium management firm is implemented, the Secretary of Defense should provide information to the public and congressional decision makers on the consortium members performing on each OTA awarded through a consortium or consortium management firm, such as by including this information in the description of requirement field in the OTA module of FPDS-Next Generation. (Recommendation 10)

DoD RESPONSE: Concur: The Department will provide instruction for users to include the names of the consortium member awardees of discrete sub-Prototype/Production OTs in the description of requirements field until planned system updates can be implemented in the FPDS OTA module.

DoD RECOMMENDATION 4: The Secretary of Defense should direct the Principal Director, Defense Pricing and Contracting, to update DOD's OTA guidance to include what agreement officers should consider when planning to use a consortium management firm to support acquisition-related activities, such as assessing the extent to which a consortium management firm is closely supporting inherently governmental functions and, for firms that do so, what enhanced management oversight activities are appropriate, if any. (Recommendation 13)

DoD RESPONSE: Concur: Defense Pricing and Contracting will provide guidance in the OT Guide update on factors the acquisition teams should consider when planning to use a consortium management firm (CMF). The guidance will address appropriate management oversight and risk mitigation procedures to be put in place to ensure inherent government functions are not performed by the CMF.

Appendix III: Comments from the Department of Health and Human Services

DEPARTMENT OF HEALTH & HUMAN SERVICES

OFFICE OF THE SECRETARY

Assistant Secretary for Legislation
Washington, DC 20201

June 29, 2021

Marie A. Mak
Director, Contracting and National Security Acquisitions
U.S. Government Accountability Office
441 G Street NW
Washington, DC 20548

Dear Ms. Mak:

Attached are comments on the U.S. Government Accountability Office's (GAO) report entitled, "*COVID-19 CONTRACTING: Actions Needed to Enhance Transparency and Oversight of Selected Awards*" (Job code 104497/GAO-21-501).

The Department appreciates the opportunity to review this report prior to publication.

Sincerely,

Jeff Hild
Acting Assistant Secretary for Legislation
Principal Deputy Assistant Secretary for Legislation

Attachment

GENERAL COMMENTS FROM THE DEPARTMENT OF HEALTH & HUMAN SERVICES ON THE GOVERNMENT ACCOUNTABILITY OFFICE'S DRAFT REPORT ENTITLED — COVID-19 CONTRACTING: ACTIONS NEEDED TO ENHANCE TRANSPARENCY AND OVERSIGHT OF SELECTED AWARDS (GAO-21-501)

The U.S. Department of Health & Human Services (HHS) appreciates the opportunity from the Government Accountability Office (GAO) to review and comment on this draft report.

Recommendation 3
The Secretary of Health and Human Services—in coordination with the change control board governing the Integrated Award Environment—should consider prioritizing the development and implementation of a systematic approach to consistently and accurately track OTAs used for national interest events and the associated dollars obligated.

HHS Response

HHS concurs with GAO's recommendation. HHS, in coordination with DoD and DHS, will submit to the IAE CCB the recommendation to prioritize the development of a systematic approach to consistently and accurately track OTAs used for national interest events and the associated dollars obligated for their implementation Government-wide.

Recommendation 8

The Secretary of Health and Human Services—in coordination with the change control board governing the Integrated Award Environment—should consider prioritizing the development and implementation of a systematic approach to track the consortium members performing for each OTA awarded through a consortium or consortium management firm.

HHS Response

HHS concurs with GAO's recommendation. HHS, in coordination with DoD and DHS, will submit to the IAE CCB the recommendation to prioritize the development of a systematic approach to track the consortium members performing for each OTA awarded through a consortium or consortium management firm for their implementation Government-wide.

Recommendation 11

Until a systematic approach to track consortium members for OTAs awarded through a consortium or consortium management firm is implemented, the Secretary of Health and Human Services should direct the Office of the Assistant Secretary for Preparedness and Response to provide information to the public and congressional decision makers on the consortium members performing on each OTA awarded through a consortium or consortium management firm, such as by including this information in the description of requirement field in the OTA module of FPDS-NG. (Recommendation 11)

HHS Response

HHS concurs with GAO's recommendation.

GENERAL COMMENTS FROM THE DEPARTMENT OF HEALTH & HUMAN SERVICES ON THE GOVERNMENT ACCOUNTABILITY OFFICE'S DRAFT REPORT ENTITLED — COVID-19 CONTRACTING: ACTIONS NEEDED TO ENHANCE TRANSPARENCY AND OVERSIGHT OF SELECTED AWARDS (GAO-21-501)

Recommendation 14

The Secretary of Health and Human Services should direct the Assistant Secretary for Preparedness and Response to update HHS's OTA guidance to include what agreement officers should consider when planning to use a consortium management firm to support acquisition-related activities, such as assessing the extent to which a consortium management firm is closely supporting inherently governmental functions and, for firms that do so, what enhanced management oversight activities are appropriate, if any. (**Recommendation 14**)

HHS Response

HHS concurs with GAO's recommendation.

Appendix IV: Comments from the Department of Homeland Security

U.S. Department of Homeland Security
Washington, DC 20528

Homeland Security

June 25, 2021

Marie A. Mak
Director, Contracting and National Security Acquisitions
U.S. Government Accountability Office
441 G Street, NW
Washington, DC 20548

Re: Management Response to Draft Report GAO-21-501, "COVID-19 CONTRACTING: Actions Needed to Enhance Transparency and Oversight of Selected Awards"

Dear Ms. Mak:

Thank you for the opportunity to comment on this draft report. The U.S. Department of Homeland Security (DHS or the Department) appreciates the U.S. Government Accountability Office's (GAO) work in planning and conducting its review and issuing this report.

The Department is pleased to note the GAO's recognition that DHS's Other Transactions (OT) policy provides for enhanced oversight of the activities consortium management firms may perform in close support of inherently governmental functions, which reduces the risk of inappropriate influence on government decisions.

DHS remains committed to, among other things: (1) procurement of vital goods and services; (2) reporting accuracy, accountability, transparency in federal spending; and (3) mitigating the potential risks associated with contractors performing acquisition support services.

The draft report contained fourteen recommendations, including four for DHS, two with which the Department concurs, and two with which we non-concur. Attached find our detailed response to each recommendation. DHS previously submitted technical comments addressing several accuracy and contextual issues under a separate cover for GAO's consideration.

Again, thank you for the opportunity to review and comment on this draft report. Please feel free to contact me if you have any questions. We look forward to working with you again in the future.

Sincerely,

JIM H CRUMPACKER
Digitally signed by JIM H CRUMPACKER
Date: 2021.06.25 07:08:32 -04'00'

JIM H. CRUMPACKER, CIA, CFE
Director
Departmental GAO-OIG Liaison Office

Attachment

Attachment: Management Response to Recommendations Contained in GAO-21-501

GAO recommended that the Secretary of Homeland Security:

Recommendation 2: In coordination with the change control board governing the Integrated Award Environment—consider prioritizing the development and implementation of a systematic approach to consistently and accurately track OTAs [Other Transaction Agreements] used for national interest events and the associated dollars obligated.

Response: Non-Concur. The DHS Office of the Chief Procurement Officer (OCPO) does not support prioritizing the development and implementation of a systematic approach to track OTAs used for national interest events and the associated dollars obligated within the Federal Procurement Data System-Next Generation (FPDS-NG). Only OTAs for research and development and prototype projects issued pursuant to 10 U.S.C. § 2371, " Research Projects: Transactions Other Than Contracts and Grants," are statutorily required to be reported in FPDS-NG, and these OTAs are rarely used in response to national interest events. Further, FPDS-NG is used to report summary level detail of awards, not dollars. Nevertheless, if there is future use of OTAs in response to a national interest event, OCPO will issue instructions on how to identify those actions when reporting to FPDS-NG is required.

DHS requests that the GAO consider this recommendation resolved and closed.

Recommendation 5: Until a systematic approach to consistently and accurately track OTAs used for national interest events is implemented, update DHS guidance to clarify how OTAs awarded in response to COVID-19 should be designated when reporting in the OTA module of FPDS-NG.

Response: Non-concur. The OCPO does not agree that additional guidance is necessary, as the designation of OTAs is already addressed in current guidance. Specifically, the FPDS-NG reporting guidance contained in the DHS Other Transactions for Research and Prototype Projects Guide, dated July 2019, (OT Guide) referenced throughout GAO's draft report is only applicable to OTAs issued pursuant to section 831 of the Homeland Security Act (HSA) of 2002, Public Law 107-296, (6 U.S.C. § 391), and does not extend to the Countering Weapons of Mass Destruction (CWMD) Office's special authority under the HSA of 2002, Public Law 107-296, § 1926 (as added by Public Law No. 115-387, § 2(a)(5), (8) (2018)) (6 U.S.C. 596(1)). Nor does the FPDS-NG reporting guidance extend to the Transportation Security Administration's (TSA's) unique OT authority under 49 U.S.C. § 106(l)(6), 114(m).

While OTAs issued pursuant to CWMD's and TSA's authorities are not required by statute to be reported in FPDS-NG, OTAs awarded pursuant to section 831 of the HSA are required, pursuant to section 874 of the Duncan Hunter National Defense Authorization Act (NDAA) for Fiscal Year 2009 (Public Law 110-417).

Accordingly, DHS included FPDS-NG reporting instructions in the OT Guide to implement section 874 of the Duncan Hunter NDAA. While the OCPO voluntarily entered all its CWMD COVID-19 OTAs into FPDS-NG in response to the public health emergency, it was not required to do so. DHS does, however, require Contracting Activities delegated with section 831 of the HSA and CWMD's OT authorities to maintain an internal OT data collection and tracking log to ensure OTAs are being documented, and that OTAs comply with statutory and policy requirements. Consequently, the current log contains information such as the identification of the awardee, the effective date, funding, and the objectives of the OTA. The DHS OCPO Office of Procurement Operations (OPO) is the only Contracting Activity authorized to execute OTAs pursuant to CWMD's OT authority. OPO has documented all the CWMD OTAs in this log and has identified them as COVID-19 related when applicable.

DHS requests that the GAO consider this recommendation resolved and closed.

Recommendation 7: In coordination with the change control board governing the Integrated Award Environment—consider prioritizing the development and implementation of a systematic approach to track the consortium members performing for each OTA awarded through a consortium or consortium management firm.

Response: Concur. In keeping with the processes of the change control board governing the Integrated Award Environment, the Department of Defense requested a change to the system to allow identification of consortia for each OTA in February 2021. The DHS OCPO will consider this change when it is brought up for governance consideration but is not yet able to identify an estimated completion date for this action, as it is dependent on the General Services Administration's governance process. Estimated Completion Date (ECD): To Be Determined.

Recommendation 12: Until a systematic approach to track consortium members for OTAs awarded through a consortium or consortium management firm is implemented across agencies, provide information to the public on the consortium members performing on each OTA awarded through a consortium or consortium management firm, such as by including this information in the description of requirement field in the OTA module of FPDS-NG.

Response: Concur. The DHS OCPO will issue a policy memorandum directing authorized Contracting Activities to identify consortium members performing OTAs in the description field of the OTA module in FPDS-NG for all OTAs that are required to be reported in the system. ECD: September 30, 2021.

Appendix V: Comments from the General Services Administration

DocuSign Envelope ID: D24C85B6-62F9-43BF-8A73-DD6E8E551026

GSA

The Administrator

June 30, 2021

The Honorable Gene L. Dodaro
Comptroller General of the United States
U.S. Government Accountability Office
Washington, DC 20548

Dear Mr. Dodaro:

The U.S. General Services Administration (GSA) appreciates the opportunity to review and comment on the draft report, "COVID-19 Contracting Actions Needed to Enhance Transparency and Oversight of Selected Awards."

In the draft report, the Government Accountability Office (GAO) issued the following recommendations to GSA:

- Recommendation 4: GAO recommends the Administrator of General Services Administration, in coordination with the change control board governing the Integrated Award Environment, should consider prioritizing the development and implementation of a systematic approach to consistently and accurately track other transaction agreements (OTA) used for national interest events and the associated dollars obligated.
- Recommendation 9: GAO recommends that the Administrator of General Services Administration, in coordination with the change control board governing the Integrated Award Environment, should consider prioritizing the development and implementation of a systematic approach to track the consortium members performing for each OTA awarded through a consortium or consortium management firm.

GSA concurs with both Recommendations 4 and 9. Recognizing that policy drives the system functionality of the Integrated Award Environment (IAE), the IAE Program Management Office (PMO), in coordination with GSA's Office of Government-wide Policy, will collaborate with executive branch stakeholders to clarify existing policy guidance on agency reporting requirements for OTAs. Following that clarification, the IAE PMO will work with the IAE Change Control Board to identify opportunities to enhance OTA tracking and reporting compliance.

If you have any additional questions or concerns, please do not hesitate to contact me or Gianelle E. Rivera, Associate Administrator, Office of Congressional and Intergovernmental Affairs, at (202) 501-0563.

Sincerely,

Katy Kale
Acting Administrator

cc: Marie A. Mak, Director, Contracting and National Security Acquisitions, GAO

U.S. General Services Administration
1800 F Street NW
Washington, DC 20405
www.gsa.gov

Appendix VI: Staff Acknowledgments

In addition to the contact named above, Penny Berrier (Assistant Director), Claire Li (Analyst in Charge), Ryan F. Braun, and Adie Lewis were principal contributors. In addition, the following people made contributions to this report: Vinayak Balasubramanian, Lorraine Ettaro, Laura Greifner, Kurt Gurka, Julia Kennon, Edward J. SanFilippo, and Roxanna T. Sun.

Chapter 3

COVID-19 Contracting: Contractor Paid Leave Reimbursements Could Provide Lessons Learned for Future Emergency Responses*

United States Government Accountability Office

Abbreviations

COVID-19	Coronavirus Disease 2019
DHS	Department of Homeland Security
DOD	Department of Defense
DOE	Department of Energy
FAR	Federal Acquisition Regulation
FPDS	Federal Procurement Data System
NASA	National Aeronautics and Space Administration
OFPP	Office of Federal Procurement Policy
OMB	Office of Management and Budget

Why GAO Did This Study

In March 2020, Congress passed the CARES Act, which provides over $2 trillion in emergency assistance for those affected by COVID-19.

* This is an edited, reformatted and augmented version of the United States Government Accountability Office Report to Congressional Addressees, Publication No. GAO-21-475, dated July 2021.

In: COVID-19 Contracting
Editor: Eric Neudorf
ISBN: 978-1-68507-710-5

Section 3610 of the CARES Act enables agencies, at their discretion, to reimburse contractors for paid leave provided to their employees and subcontractors who are unable to access work sites due to facility closures or other restrictions, and whose duties cannot be performed remotely during the pandemic. The CARES Act also includes a provision for GAO to review federal contracting pursuant to authorities provided in the Act.

In September 2020, GAO found that agencies had not made much use of section 3610 authority as of July 2020, and expectations of future use varied.

This report (1) examines how selected federal agencies have used section 3610 authority and (2) presents selected contractors' perspectives on COVID-19 paid leave reimbursement. GAO reviewed guidance and data and interviewed cognizant officials from four agencies with contract obligations greater than $10 billion in fiscal year 2019. GAO also selected a non-generalizable sample of 15 contractors that received or requested section 3610 reimbursements from one or more of the selected agencies and conducted semi-structured interviews of contractor representatives.

What GAO Recommends

OMB should collect and share lessons learned from federal agencies' implementation of COVID-19 paid leave reimbursement. OMB concurred with this recommendation.

What GAO Found

To help government contractors keep their workforce in a ready state during the COVID-19 pandemic, section 3610 of the CARES Act generally authorized government agencies to reimburse contractors for paid leave provided to contractor personnel and subcontractors during the national emergency. Section 3610 did not appropriate specific funding for this purpose. The four agencies GAO reviewed—the Departments of Defense, Energy, and Homeland Security, and NASA—reported use of section 3610 authority totaling at least $882.8 million over 14 months. The extent to which the agencies used the authority varied, from $1.4 million at Homeland Security to $760.7 million at Energy.

Further, Defense officials estimated that defense contractors have more than $4 billion in paid leave costs that are potentially eligible for reimbursement under section 3610. Defense officials also noted, however, that the department does not plan to reimburse this full amount using existing funding. Agencies also based their reimbursement decisions on the nature of the work performed by contractors, such as whether telework was an option.

Twelve out of the 15 contractors GAO interviewed reported that paid leave reimbursement had a great or moderate effect on their ability to retain employees (see figure), in particular those with specialized skills or clearances.

Selected Contractors' Views on the Effect of Paid Leave Reimbursement on Workforce Retention

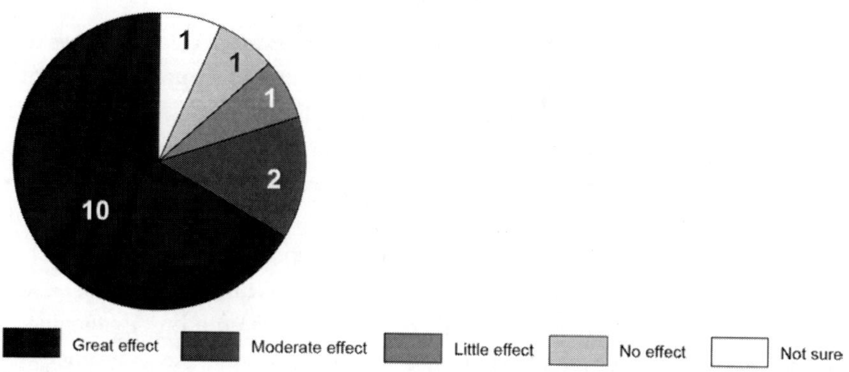

Source: GAO analysis of contractor representative interview responses. | GAO-21-475.

Given the urgency of the pandemic, agencies prioritized quick implementation of section 3610 over a more deliberative process, resulting in variations such as how agencies tracked use of the authority. Officials from all four agencies said that they either have captured or intend to capture lessons learned from implementing section 3610 and are willing to share these with other federal agencies. However, the Office of Management and Budget (OMB)—which coordinates government-wide contracting policy—has not collected and shared lessons learned. With coordination from OMB's Office of Federal Procurement Policy, the government could seize an opportunity to enhance implementation of paid leave reimbursement provisions that may be enacted as part of rapid federal responses to future emergencies.

July 28, 2021
Congressional Addressees

The Coronavirus Disease 2019 (COVID-19) pandemic has resulted in catastrophic loss of life and substantial damage to the global economy, stability, and security. On March 11, 2020, the World Health Organization characterized COVID-19 as a pandemic, and 2 days later the U.S. President declared COVID-19 a national emergency. In response to this unprecedented global crisis, in March 2020 Congress passed, and the President signed into law, the CARES Act, which provided over $2 trillion in emergency assistance and health care response for individuals, families, and businesses affected by COVID-19.[1]

The CARES Act included a provision for GAO to provide a comprehensive audit and review of federal contracting pursuant to authorities provided in the Act.[2] Section 3610 of the CARES Act generally permits federal agencies to reimburse contractors who provide paid leave to their employees and subcontractors who are unable to access work sites due to facility closures and other restrictions and who cannot telework during the COVID-19 pandemic. This authority currently applies through September 30, 2021, following a number of extensions. While authorizing such reimbursements, Congress did not appropriate specific funding to agencies to cover these expenses. Rather, it allowed agencies to use funding made available by the CARES Act or any other act. In September 2020, we reported on section 3610 implementation guidance issued by selected agencies, as well as the extent to which those agencies reported use of the authority.[3]

---

[1] Pub. L. No. 116-136, 134 Stat. 281 (2020). As of March 31, 2021, laws that make appropriations or provide some other relief in response to the COVID-19 pandemic include: the American Rescue Plan Act of 2021, Pub. L. No. 117-2, 135 Stat. 4 (2021); the Consolidated Appropriations Act, 2021, Pub. L. No. 116-260, 134 Stat. 1182 (2020); the Paycheck Protection Program and Health Care Enhancement Act, Pub. L. No. 116-139, 134 Stat. 620 (2020); the Families First Coronavirus Response Act, Pub. L. No. 116-127, 134 Stat. 178 (2020); and the Coronavirus Preparedness and Response Supplemental Appropriations Act, 2020, Pub. L. No. 116-123, 134 Stat. 146 (2020).

[2] We regularly issue government-wide reports on the federal response to COVID-19. For the latest report, see GAO, *COVID-19: Continued Attention Needed to Enhance Federal Preparedness, Response, Service Delivery, and Program Integrity*, GAO-21-551 (Washington, D.C.: July 19, 2021). Our next government-wide report will be issued in October 2021 and will be available on GAO's website at https://www.gao.gov/coronavirus.

[3] GAO, *COVID-19 Contracting: Observations on Contractor Paid Leave Reimbursement Guidance and Use*, GAO-20-662 (Washington, D.C.: Sept. 3, 2020).

This report (1) examines how selected federal agencies have used section 3610 authority and (2) presents selected contractors' perspectives on COVID-19 paid leave reimbursement.

To examine how selected federal agencies have used section 3610 authority, we identified the seven federal agencies with contract obligations greater than $10 billion in fiscal year 2019. We reviewed these agencies' use of section 3610 authority as of July 20, 2020, as reported to the Federal Procurement Data System (FPDS), and selected the three agencies with reported use. These three agencies were the Department of Defense (DOD), Department of Energy (DOE), and the National Aeronautics and Space Administration (NASA). As a point of comparison, we also selected one agency—the Department of Homeland Security (DHS)—that had not reported use of section 3610 authority as of July 20, 2020. For these four agencies, we gathered and analyzed guidance regarding section 3610 and data on its use either collected by agencies or reported to FPDS from January 31, 2020, through March 31, 2021; and interviewed or received written responses from cognizant agency officials.[4] We also interviewed officials from the Office of Management and Budget's (OMB) Office of Federal Procurement Policy (OFPP) due to this agency's role in coordinating government-wide contracting policy. To assess the reliability of data from agencies and FPDS, we reviewed related documentation, such as data validation rules, and interviewed knowledgeable agency officials. We determined the data were sufficiently reliable for the purposes of describing the extent to which selected agencies reported use of section 3610 authority.

To identify selected contractors' perspectives on COVID-19 paid leave reimbursement, we selected a non-generalizable sample of 15 prime contractors that, according to agency data, have received or requested section 3610 reimbursements from one or more agencies in this review.

We selected contractors to reflect a range of company sizes, ownership structures, and product and service offerings. We conducted semi- structured interviews of cognizant contractor representatives about their experiences seeking reimbursement from different agencies and reviewed available company financial information. We also interviewed representatives from

[4] According to the General Services Administration, FPDS is the federal government's authoritative source for contract data. Contracts whose estimated value is $10,000 or more are reported to FPDS, as well as every modification to those contracts, regardlessof dollar value. On October 17, 2020, the FPDS reports module was retired and the https://SAM.gov Data Bank is now the only place to create and run both standard and ad hoc reports on federal contract data.

industry associations about contractors' experiences seeking reimbursement from different agencies, and about why some contractors have not requested reimbursements. Additionally, we interviewed or received written responses from cognizant representatives from four contractors identified as having not yet requested section 3610 reimbursements from agencies in our review at the time of selection. See appendix I for more information on our objectives, scope, and methodology, including a listing of the contractors and industry associations that participated in this review.

We conducted this performance audit from October 2020 to July 2021 in accordance with generally accepted government auditing standards.

Those standards require that we plan and perform the audit to obtain sufficient, appropriate evidence to provide a reasonable basis for our findings and conclusions based on our audit objectives. We believe that the evidence obtained provides a reasonable basis for our findings and conclusions based on our audit objectives.

Background

Contracting Responses to COVID-19

The CARES Act was enacted on March 27, 2020. Section 3610 generally authorizes federal agencies to reimburse contractors for paid leave provided to a contractor's employees and subcontractors who are unable to access work sites due to facility closures or other restrictions, and whose duties cannot be performed remotely during the COVID-19 pandemic. This authority originally applied through September 30, 2020, but was subsequently extended until December 11, 2020, then March 31, 2021, and then again through September 30, 2021.[5] While authorizing such reimbursements, section 3610 did not appropriate any additional funding to agencies to cover these expenses. Use of this authority is at the government's discretion and not mandatory, a point emphasized in implementation guidance subsequently issued by OMB and selected agencies. Several industry associations had advocated for prior extensions of section 3610 authority as well as for supplemental funding for section 3610 reimbursements.

---

[5] Pub. L. No. 116-136, 134 Stat. 281, § 3610; Continuing Appropriations Act, 2021, and Other Extensions Act, Pub. L. No. 116-159, 134 Stat. 709, § 140 (2020); Pub. L. No. 116-260, 134 Stat. 1182, § 1002; Pub. L. No. 117-2, 135 Stat. 4, § 4015.

While not the focus of this report, the federal government took other steps to support contractors during the pandemic. For example, to help companies manage cash flow, DOD increased progress payment rates.[6] Congress also made additional financial relief available through the Paycheck Protection Program, designed to provide loans for small businesses to keep their workers on payroll, and included in the CARES Act an employee retention tax credit for businesses.[7]

Contract Costs

Federal agency contract spending on products and services in fiscal year 2020 totaled over $660 billion. DOD is responsible for almost two-thirds of this amount, for services including professional engineering/technical services and general health care, and for products including fixed wing aircraft, combat ships, and landing vessels. Civilian agencies contract for various services, including professional services and maintenance and security of their buildings, and acquire products such as information technology hardware and software. Federal agencies typically contract with private-sector companies to acquire these products and services.

The price of a contract typically consists of various elements such as the cost of materials, labor costs, and profit or fee. Contractors' labor costs include the costs of paid leave such as sick leave, holidays, and vacations. These costs are generally considered fringe benefits and may be reimbursed on certain contracts to the extent that they are reasonable and are required by law, employer-employee agreement, or an established policy of the contractor. These indirect costs are typically spread across multiple contracts at a particular contractor business division, as opposed to direct costs such as the

---

[6] Through progress payments, DOD can finance certain contractor expenses as work progresses, including financing payments made to subcontractors. Contract financing assists the contractor in managing expenses such as material, labor, and overhead. Progress payments based on costs are determined as a percentage of the costs incurred by the contractor. Prior to the pandemic, DOD paid 80 percent of incurred costs of large businesses and 90 percent of incurred costs of small businesses. However, in responseto COVID-19, in March 2020 DOD increased the customary progress payment rates for eligible contractors to 90 percent for large businesses and 95 percent for small businesses. GAO has ongoing work regarding DOD's use of the increased rate of progress payments during the COVID-19 national emergency. For additional information on progress payments, see GAO, *Contract Financing: DOD Should Comprehensively Assess How Its Policies Affect the Defense Industry*, GAO-19-406 (Washington, D.C.: June 27, 2019).

[7] Pub. L. No. 116-136, §§ 1102, 1106, 2301; 85 Fed. Reg. 20811, 20814 (Apr. 15, 2020).

labor and material costs that can be associated with and allocated to a specific contract.[8]

Prior GAO and Agency Offices of Inspector General Reports on Section 3610

In September 2020, we reported that, in general, agencies had not made much use of section 3610 authority to reimburse contractor paid leave costs as of July 2020. Agencies' expectations of future requests from contractors varied and depended on factors including availability of funding.[9] We also found that, in several instances, agencies identified other contracting authorities that could be used in place of or in addition to section 3610. For example, DHS guidance identified certain standard Federal Acquisition Regulation (FAR) clauses through which equitable adjustments to contract prices in response to COVID-19 disruptions could be made.[10] Similarly, NASA guidance identified some existing FAR and NASA FAR Supplement clauses through which the agency could reimburse paid leave costs.[11] DOD guidance outlined additional ways to address the effect of COVID-19 on contractors, including the possibility of relief from contract delivery requirements in the event of delays caused by COVID-19, and contract modifications, subject to the availability of funds, to reflect changes to the government's needs. OMB advised agencies to report contract modifications using section 3610 authority to FPDS, using terminology provided by OMB. However, in that same report, we found that not all agencies' section 3610 reimbursements were reported to FPDS as such. For example, DOE officials told us they did not need to issue a contract modification to obligate additional funding for paid leave reimbursement.

Offices of Inspector General at several agencies have reported on or are assessing the implementation of section 3610. For example, in December

---

8 Depending on an agency's guidance, there may be an option to request reimbursement for section 3610 paid leave directly against a contract, but there may also be opportunities for reimbursement across multiple contracts as part of a global settlement process. For instance, we previously reported that DOD's guidance tailored the reimbursement request process to the circumstances of the contractor, depending on whether it seeks reimbursement in relation to a single contract, multiple contracts, or at the level of an entire business unit. GAO-20-662.

9 GAO-20-662.

10 FAR § 52.243-1 (Changes-Fixed-Price) and FAR § 52.243-2 (Changes-Cost- Reimbursement).

11 Cited authorities include FAR § 52.242-15 (Stop-Work Order) and NASA FAR Supplement § 1852.242-72 (Denied Access to NASA Facilities).

2020, the DOD Office of Inspector General found that contracting officers had to rely on contractors to self-certify that the section 3610 costs they claimed were the only reimbursements the contractors received for paid leave, and that the contractors were not receiving reimbursements for the same expenses from any other sources.[12] In January 2021, the Office of Inspector General of the National Reconnaissance Office also completed an evaluation of that agency's implementation of section 3610.[13] According to officials, the Offices of Inspector General of NASA and DOE are also undertaking work related to section 3610.

Agencies Varied in Their Use of Section 3610 Authority and Prioritized Implementation Speed over a More Deliberative Process

The four agencies we reviewed made use of section 3610 authority to varying degrees, identifying a total of at least $882.8 million in paid leave costs incurred by their contractors over 14 months, which the agencies either had reimbursed or were assessing for potential reimbursement.

The agencies tracked this use via different methods. Further, the agencies based their decisions to use this authority on the type of work performed by contractors and assessments of their own funding priorities. Agencies' implementation of section 3610 was also shaped by the extent to which they had existing processes for addressing costs claimed by contractors. In implementing this authority, and given the urgent need to respond quickly to the pandemic, agencies prioritized speed over a more deliberative process.

Extent to Which Selected Agencies Used Section 3610 Authority Varied

The four agencies we reviewed—DOD, DOE, DHS, and NASA—identified at least $882.8 million in section 3610 paid leave costs incurred by their

[12] Department of Defense, Office of Inspector General, Audit of Department of Defense Implementation of Section 3610 of the Coronavirus Aid, Relief, and Economic Security Act, DODIG-2021-030 (Alexandria, VA: Dec. 9, 2020).

[13] National Reconnaissance Office, Office of Inspector General, Evaluation of the National Reconnaissance Office's Implementation of Section 3610 Authorized by the Coronavirus Aid, Relief, and Economic Security Act, Project Number 2020-004 S (Chantilly, VA: Jan. 4, 2021).

contractors from January 31, 2020, through March 31, 2021, which the agencies either had reimbursed or were assessing for potential reimbursement. The amount of use varied greatly by agency (see table 1).

Table 1. Use of Section 3610 Authority as reported by selected agencies from January 31, 2020 through March 31, 2021

Agency	Use of section 3610 authority (millions of dollars)
Department of Energy[a]	760.7
Department of Defense	73.2
National Aeronautics and Space Administration (NASA)[b]	At least 47.5
Department of Homeland Security	1.4

Source: GAO analysis of Federal Procurement Data System and agency-reported data. | GAO-21-475.

[a] The amount reported by the Department of Energy represents potential section 3610 costs incurred by contractors (e.g., invoiced amounts), unlike amounts reported by the Departments of Defense and Homeland Security which were based on obligations reported to the Federal Procurement Data System.

[b] As of March 31, 2021, NASA reported $80 million in potential section 3610 reimbursements in its internal invoice payment tracking system since March 2020. However, a NASA official stated that this amount includes both section 3610 and non-section 3610 costs related to COVID-19, and based on initial assessments the amount for section 3610 costs is at least $47.5 million. A NASA official noted that contracting officers will manually separate these costs when closing contractors' requests for equitable adjustment in response to the pandemic and, at that point, will have more visibility into the agency's use of section 3610 to reimburse contractors' paid leave costs.

Agencies Used Different Ways to Track Use of Section 3610

The agencies in our review tracked the use of section 3610 in a variety of ways—including in FPDS per OMB guidance and via tracking mechanisms established by the agencies themselves—and captured different types of data. OMB's April 2020 guidance noted that, to track the use of section 3610, agencies should report contract modifications allowing payments authorized by section 3610 to FPDS by entering "COVID-19 3610" at the beginning of the Description of Requirements field. We found some differences between the amounts publicly reported in FPDS and internally tracked by agencies.[14] Specifically:

- At the headquarters level, DHS tracked its use of section 3610 through obligations reported by contracting officers in FPDS. DHS officials noted that these records sometimes included non-section 3610 obligations, and that they periodically reviewed and corrected such instances.
- In the case of DOE, the agency's internal data showed $760.7 million in potential section 3610 costs incurred by contractors as of March 31, 2021, in comparison to the $357.9 million in section 3610 obligations reported in FPDS as of the same date. DOE officials said that the agency was able to use existing contract obligations to cover section 3610 costs incurred by contractors; as such, officials said DOE did not require issuing new contract modifications to add funding. Such modifications would have needed to be reported in FPDS pursuant to OMB's guidance. For tracking purposes, DOE officials told us the agency incorporated special coding into its invoicing and payment systems for expenditures related to COVID-19 since FPDS is not designed to collect this type of spend information. DOE officials also noted that the amounts tracked by the agency as costs incurred by contractors do not necessarily equate to actual or final reimbursements made to contractors, as reimbursements are provisional under cost-reimbursement contracts and will be finalized by DOE after they have been audited.
- In the case of DOD, the amount originally reported in FPDS exceeded the amount the agency internally tracked. DOD reported in FPDS that it had obligated $91.3 million in section 3610-related obligations as of March 31, 2021, whereas DOD officials stated that, upon reviewing the reported information, the actual amount was $73.2 million. As we reported in September 2020, these reviews identified instances in which obligations reported in FPDS as uses of section 3610 authority actually reflected a combination of section 3610 and non-section 3610 obligations, such as for general services or test operations. Officials from DOD's Defense Pricing and Contracting

[14] Agencies in our review did not centrally track use of other authorities to reimburse contractors for paid leave costs, such as FAR-based contract clauses, although officials noted that it was possible that contracting officers were using such authorities.

office told us they continue to review FPDS records for obligations using section 3610 authority to check that they are accurately coded and meet DOD's section 3610 policy requirements.

- At NASA, the agency reported $11.1 million in FPDS as section 3610 obligations as of March 31, 2021, but NASA officials said that they do not use FPDS for the purpose of tracking use of section 3610 authority. Rather, NASA uses an invoice payment tracking system to monitor its use of the authority, which, as of March 31, 2021, showed $80 million in potential section 3610 reimbursements since March 2020. However, a NASA official told us that this amount includes both section 3610 and non-section 3610 costs related to COVID-19; based on initial assessments, the amount for section 3610 costs is at least $47.5 million. A NASA official said that contracting officers will manually separate these costs when closing contractors' requests for equitable adjustment in response to the pandemic and, at that point, will have more visibility into NASA's use of section 3610.

Agencies' Decisions to Use Section 3610 Authority Were Based Largely on Type of Work and Funding Priorities

Agency officials told us their decisions to use section 3610 authority to reimburse contractor paid leave depended, in part, on the type of work contractors performed—specifically, the extent to which (1) contractor employees could not be onsite due to facility closures and (2) teleworking was not feasible. Such circumstances included when contractor employees needed to work with classified information or were helping test or produce an item, such as an aircraft or ship, but could not access a facility due to restrictions associated with COVID-19. In such cases, reimbursements for paid leave would keep employees—who might have security clearances or key technical knowledge and skills required to support the agency's mission—in a ready state able to return to work quickly and reduce the chance of these employees leaving the contractor.

A related factor that may have affected facility accessibility—and thus the potential need to use section 3610—was the identification by DHS in March 2020 of personnel considered essential critical infrastructure workers during the COVID-19 response.[15] This step established the expectation that workers in critical infrastructure sectors—including contractor and subcontractor personnel—would maintain their normal work schedules while following federal, state, and local safety guidelines. The defense industrial base was identified as a critical infrastructure sector, increasing the likelihood that contractors in this sector would continue operations and limit their need to place employees on paid leave.

Agencies in our review also generally based their decisions to use section 3610 authority to reimburse contractors for paid leave on an assessment of funding priorities. For example:

- NASA officials told us that the agency decided to use existing funding for paid leave reimbursements to maintain the space industrial base and retain contractors' technical skill sets because this approach would lessen the effect on the agency's missions. NASA officialsadded that doing so allowed the agency to continue to make progress on missions including the Mars Exploration Program. In addition to existing funding, NASA received $60 million in supplemental appropriations in the CARES Act to prevent, prepare for, and respond to COVID-19. According to NASA officials, $5.2 million of this amount helped fund contractors' paid leave reimbursements, while the remainder supported additional information technology needs due to increased telework, increased cleaning and personal protective equipment, and other activities. NASA officials told us that they may request additional supplemental appropriations from Congress to support costs that could include, but would not be limited to, funding paid leave reimbursements.
- DOE officials stated that the agency used existing funding to reimburse contractors for paid leave costs because it was in the government's best interest to retain specialized staff, such as

[15] DHS's Cybersecurity and Infrastructure Security Agency is responsible for providing strategic guidance to ensure security and resilience of national critical infrastructure. Homeland Security Act of 2002, Pub. L. No. 107-296, 116 Stat. 2135 (2002), as amended by the Cybersecurity and Infrastructure Security Agency Act of 2018, Pub. L. No. 115-278, 132 Stat. 4168 (2018). As a result, this agency developed a list of essential critical infrastructure workers to inform community decision-making and assist in prioritizing efforts. However, the list is advisory and not a federal directive. The defense industrial base is defined as the worldwide industrial complex that enables research, development, design, production, delivery, and maintenance of military weapons systems/software systems, subsystems, and components or parts as well as purchased services to meet U.S. military requirements.

contractor employees who work in the agency's National Laboratories or those who are under contract to help remediate nuclear waste sites.[16]

- Although DOD has used existing funding to reimburse $73.2 million in paid leave costs, this is a small portion of the total amount it estimates it needed to reimburse contractors' paid leave costs. In December 2020, DOD notified Congress that it estimated contractors across the defense industrial base had incurred $4.25 billion in paid leave costs potentially eligible for reimbursement under section 3610. This amount—equivalent to 1.5 percent of DOD's total contract obligations across the same period—was based on rough order of magnitude estimates through December 11, 2020, which were provided by DOD's largest contractors and extrapolated across its industrial base.
- DOD officials told us that, with the extension of section 3610 authority through September 30, 2021, DOD contractors will likely incur additional costs for providing paid leave to their employees. According to DOD officials, DOD's current estimate for section 3610 paid leave costs across the defense industrial base from March 27, 2020, to September 30, 2021, is $7 billion. DOD officials noted that section 3610 authorized, but did not appropriate, funds for reimbursements.
- They added that while DOD might be able to use other appropriated funds to reimburse contractors, it would not be able to do so without jeopardizing modernization or readiness efforts.[17] Representatives of several large contractors told us that they would not go through the effort of putting together all the information DOD requires in support of reimbursement requests until they had a clearer indication that

---

16 DOE officials noted that DOE and the National Nuclear Security Administration—a semi-autonomous agency within DOE—continue to see a downward trend of costs requested for reimbursement that are allowed under section 3610, and that they would seek an extension of the authority beyond September 30, 2021, should conditions warrant.

17 DOD also notified Congress that it estimates needing an additional $6.55 billion to reimburse contractors for other COVID-19-related costs, including the purchase of personal protective equipment, increased cleaning, and the costs of reconfiguring facilities and offices to support social distancing. DOD officials stated that the agency has sought a total of $13.6 billion in supplemental appropriations from Congress to fund all COVID-19- related costs through fiscal year 2023. This amount takes into account cost reductions due to COVID-19 such as decreased travel costs.

DOD had funding it was prepared to use for this purpose.[18] In addition, two of the contractors in our review stated in recent financial report filings that they may not be able to fully recover paid leave costs under fixed- price-type contracts. DOD officials noted the possibility that, to the extent that paid leave costs—particularly on fixed-price-type contracts—are not reimbursed, contractors might increase indirect cost rates on future contracts.[19]

- DHS officials cited the agency's ability to find ways to keep facilities open, as well as keep contractors working, as reasons for its relatively low level of paid leave reimbursement. For example, while increased telework reduced the need for frequent building cleaning, DHS modified contracts so that cleaning contractors performed more thorough cleaning. DHS officials said this enabled the contractors to keep working, helped meet DHS's requirement to have facilities available when needed, and readied facilities for eventual full reopening. As of March 2021, DHS officials said that they do not plan to seek supplemental appropriations for paid leave costs.

Existing Processes Informed How Agencies Implemented Section 3610

The extent to which agencies had existing processes for addressing costs claimed by contractors also informed how they approached implementation of section 3610.

- In NASA's case, prior to the COVID-19 pandemic, the agency identified in existing contractual clauses contractor responsibilities and contracting officer authorities in the event that work could not be safely performed at contractor facilities, or if a NASA facility was

---

[18] A statement from a senior DOD official indicated that global settlements at the business unit or corporate level—as provided for in guidance issued by DOD in August 2020— rather than on a contract-by-contract basis, may be the preferred approach for reimbursing its largest contractors should funding be available.

[19] Defense Contract Audit Agency officials noted they anticipated seeing COVID-19 effects, including paid leave, reflected in contractors' incurred cost submissions due the summer of 2021, as well as in forward pricing rate proposals. Contractor forward pricing rate proposals are part of the negotiation of forward pricing rate agreements with contracting officers which establish rates used as bases for contract pricing during the period covered by the agreement. FAR §15.407-3; FAR subpart 42.17.

closed and there was no work the contractor could accomplish from a remote location.[20] Circumstances that might temporarily close a NASA facility include natural disasters such as hurricanes. For example, NASA includes a standard FAR clause governing stop-work orders, which states that the contracting officer shall make an equitable adjustment to a contract's price or delivery schedule, or both, should certain conditions be met. Additionally, a unique NASA clause states that the contracting officer may consider making an equitable adjustment or other remedy to compensate for the period that NASA facilities were not accessible to contractor employees. NASA's guidance for section 3610 notes that the CARES Act complements the agency's existing authorities. To achieve a standard agency-wide approach to implement these clauses, NASA established advance agreements—incorporated into contracts through bilateral modifications—that identified how to treat costs associated with employees unable to work remotely.[21] For example, the advance agreements provide instructions for billing and labeling the invoice to reflect COVID-19 terminology and require separation on the invoice of labor and non-labor expenses. NASA officials said that the advance agreements fostered communication between contracting officers and contractors and established a clear process for requesting and receiving paid leave reimbursements under section 3610.

- DOD implemented section 3610, in part, by issuing a class deviation to the FAR and Defense Federal Acquisition Regulation Supplementthat established a new cost principle.[22] This class deviation established the allowability of section 3610 costs.[23] Paid

[20] FAR § 52.242-15 (Stop-Work Order) and NASA FAR Supplement § 1852.242-72 (Denied Access to NASA Facilities).

[21] FAR § 43.103(a) (Types of contract modifications). A bilateral modification is a contract modification that is signed by the contractor and the contracting officer, and its uses include making negotiated equitable adjustments resulting from the issuance of a change order. A unilateral modification, on the other hand, is a contract modification that is signed only by the contracting officer.

[22] DOD Class Deviation 2020-O0013, Rev. 4 (March 23, 2021). See also DOD Class Deviation 2020-O0021, Rev. 3 (March 23, 2021). Class deviations are deviations from the FAR necessary to meet the specific needs and requirements of an agency, and which affect more than one contract action. FAR §§ 1.402, 1.404. Class deviations are also issued in relation to agency acquisition regulations; for example, they allow DOD organizations to deviate from the Defense Federal Acquisition Regulation Supplement. Defense Federal Acquisition Regulation Supplement subpart 201.4.

[23] DOD Class Deviation 2020-O0013, Rev. 4 (March 23, 2021). See also DOD Class Deviation 2020-O0021, Rev. 3 (March 23, 2021). Class deviations are deviations from the FAR

leave reimbursement remains at the discretion of the contracting officer, who is expected to consider the immediacy of the contractor's need for financial relief. For example, some contractors may still have incoming revenue and be able to conduct work remotely, whereas others may be unable to conduct any business and have difficulties making payroll and retaining employees.

- According to DHS guidance for implementing section 3610, DHS's contracting officers can negotiate bilateral contract modifications to support contractors' needs in order to maintain a ready state. More specifically, according to the guidance, DHS's modifications require the contractor to agree to segregate and report the actual costs of the leave payments for each employee. DHS officials said that they developed this process because contracting officers are familiar with using bilateral modifications, allowing them to quickly implement section 3610.
- According to DOE officials, paid leave costs are allowable if they meet applicable FAR requirements; therefore, no special authorities were needed to recognize paid leave costs as reimbursable under contracts. DOE officials said that the agency generally used existing processes to review and approve paid leave reimbursement requests. For example, according to DOE officials, under the department's existing processes, requests for paid leave reimbursements are provisional under cost-reimbursement contracts and will be finalized by DOE after they have been audited. The officials stated that program officials and contracting officers have significant discretion in deciding how to implement paid leave reimbursements, including through means such as contract modifications and advance agreements. For example, DOE officials noted that one program established advance agreements to address which costs the government would consider reasonable for reimbursement. However, DOE did not require the use of advance agreements because such a step might not be necessary in some cases when implementing section 3610, according to officials. Further, DOE officials expressed cost accounting standards-related concerns about contractors charging

---

necessary to meet the specific needs and requirements of an agency, and which affect more than one contract action. FAR §§ 1.402, 1.404. Class deviations are also issued in relation to agency acquisition regulations; for example, they allow DOD organizations to deviate from the Defense Federal Acquisition Regulation Supplement. Defense Federal Acquisition Regulation Supplement subpart 201.4.

COVID-19 paid leave to affected contracts as a direct cost instead of an indirect cost. DOE officials also observed that large- scale changes to agreed-upon cost accounting practices can take considerable time to coordinate with contracting officers and can have significant effects on costs across different contract types at multiple federal agencies.

Agencies Prioritized Quick Implementation; Opportunities Exist to Collect and Share Lessons Learned

Given the urgency associated with responding to the pandemic and mitigating its effect on contractors' ability to support their government customers, agency officials told us they prioritized implementation speed over a more deliberative process. Overall, each of the agencies in our review—as well as OMB—issued initial guidance outlining how they planned to implement section 3610 and the extent to which they would use or adapt existing mechanisms. While some coordination across and within agencies occurred following enactment of section 3610, our September 2020 report found a number of inconsistencies between different agencies' initial guidance documents, such as the start date for reimbursement of section 3610 paid leave costs.

Furthermore, several of the contractors in our review work with multiple agencies, and they observed variations in how agencies implemented section 3610. For example, several contractor representatives noted that NASA's process to reimburse contractors affected by COVID-19 was a clearer pathway to reimbursement than DOD's approach. Finally, as noted above, the ways that agencies tracked use of section 3610 relied on different data sources and required manual adjustments for accuracy, adding to the challenges of obtaining information on use of section 3610.

In prior work, we found that the collecting and sharing of lessons learned from previous programs or projects provides organizations with a powerful method for sharing ideas for improving work processes.[24] In particular, we

---

[24] GAO, Grants Management: OMB Should Collect and Share Lessons Learned from Use of COVID-19-Related Grant Flexibilities, GAO-21-318 (Washington, D.C.: Mar. 31, 2021); DOD Utilities Privatization: Improved Data Collection and Lessons Learned Archive Could Help Reduce Time to Award Contracts, GAO-20-104 (Washington, D.C.: Apr. 2, 2020); Project Management: DOE and NNSA Should Improve Their Lessons-Learned Process for Capital Asset Projects, GAO-19-25 (Washington, D.C.: Dec. 21, 2018); and

found that collecting and sharing lessons learned from an interagency effort is valuable since one agency can share its experiences with other agencies that may benefit from the information.[25] Furthermore, organizations that identify and apply lessons learned can ensure they factor beneficial information into planning for future efforts and limit the recurrence of challenges that can be anticipated in advance. We have previously reported on actions Congress and OMB have taken to strengthen agencies' use of evidence about whether federal programs and activities achieve intended results in planning future efforts. For example, the Foundations for Evidence-Based Policymaking Act of 2018 requires major federal agencies to develop learning agendas.[26]

Officials from all four agencies in our review said that they either have captured or intend to capture lessons learned from the implementation of section 3610 and would be willing to share these with other federal agencies. However, OMB—which coordinates government-wide contracting policy among other responsibilities—has not collected and shared agencies' lessons learned. With coordination from OFPP within OMB, such information could help OMB and agencies to enhance the implementation of any new paid leave reimbursement provisions that may be enacted as part of rapid federal responses to future emergencies.

Contractors Cited Workforce Retention as the Main Benefit of Paid Leave Reimbursement

The primary benefit of section 3610 paid leave reimbursement cited by contractors in our review was its effect on workforce retention, in particular for workers with specialized skills or clearances. Contractor representatives noted that they took other steps to mitigate the effect of COVID-19 prior to seeking paid leave reimbursement, leading to fewer individuals being placed on paid leave.

Federal Real Property Security: Interagency Security Committee Should Implement a Lessons- Learned Process, GAO-12-901 (Washington, D.C.: Sept. 10, 2012).

[25] GAO-12-901.

[26] For more information on developing learning agendas, see GAO, *Evidence-Based Policymaking: Selected Agencies Coordinate Activities, but Could Enhance Collaboration*, GAO-20-119 (Washington, D.C.: Dec. 4, 2019).

Contractors Cited Workforce Retention as Primary Benefit of Section 3610

Contractor representatives noted that the availability of paid leave reimbursement under section 3610 reinforced workforce retention by boosting employee morale, allowing employees to maintain health benefits and paychecks during a time of uncertainty, and increasing safety by encouraging possibly sick employees to stay at home.

Contractor representatives stated they were generally supportive of section 3610 to reimburse paid leave costs, noting that its use allowed them to avoid some furloughs or layoffs, retain key skill sets in high demand, and keep employees in a ready state able to quickly remobilize to support the government (see figure 1).

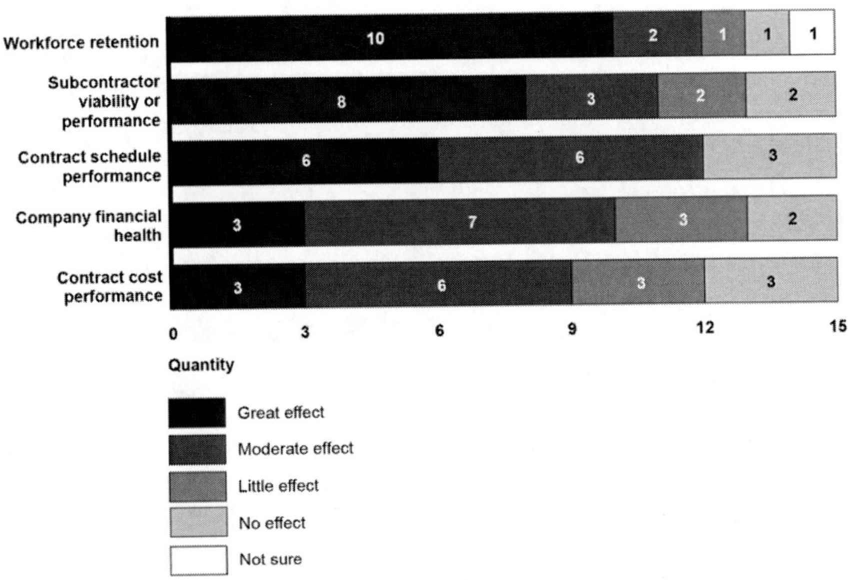

Source: GAO analysis of contractor representative interview responses. | GAO-21-475.

Figure 1. Effects of Section 3610 Paid Leave Reimbursement Cited by Contractors GAO Reviewed.

Contractors we spoke with cited the ability to retain employees with specialized skills or clearances in their decisions to seek paid leave reimbursement on particular contracts. For example, representatives of one contractor stated that receiving section 3610 reimbursement eased the fear of permanently losing employees with years of training and experience, and representatives of another contractor noted the ability to keep employees with security clearances due to paid leave reimbursement.[27]

In addition to employee retention, contractors noted other benefits associated with receiving section 3610 reimbursements:

- Contractors noted the effect of section 3610 reimbursement on the ability of subcontractors—sometimes also small businesses—to remain viable and able to perform. As representatives of one contractor noted, small businesses do not always have access to the same financial resources as larger businesses, so a missed payment could have a significant effect on their viability. However, by being able to submit invoices and receive payment under normal timelines, these subcontractors could retain their personnel and remain financially healthy.
- Representatives for some DOD contractors noted a contract cost accounting benefit of section 3610. Paid leave is usually a fringe benefit allocated as an indirect cost across multiple contracts. However, DOD's section 3610 guidance allows for COVID-19 paid leave costs to be charged directly to affected contracts.[28] For example, one contractor's representative noted that if the contractor had to treat these as indirect costs, it would have had a potentially significant effect on rate structures and increased future contract prices.

---

[27] We have previously noted extensive challenges with the timely processing of personnel security clearances across the federal government and, in 2018, GAO added the government-wide personnel security clearance process to the High-Risk List due to its various challenges. See GAO, *High-Risk Series: Dedicated Leadership Needed to Address Limited Progress in Most High-Risk Areas*, GAO-21-119SP (Washington, D.C.: Mar. 2, 2021).

[28] DOD recommended that contractors charge section 3610 costs to a newly created cost category, "Other Direct Costs COVID-19", while recognizing that in some situations, it may be more appropriate to charge these costs through indirect cost pools. DOD noted that, by creating a new category of costs, contractors may avoid any potential issues with disclosed accounting policies and procedures, cost accounting standards, or their cost accounting standards disclosure statements.

Contractors Used Other Approaches to Mitigate the Effect of COVID-19 and the Need to Place Employees on Paid Leave

Our review of contractor financial statements and discussions with contractor representatives indicated that contractors took a variety of steps to keep employees and subcontractors working to the extent possible and, from their perspectives, minimized the need to seek reimbursement for paid leave costs. For example, in addition to following Centers for Disease Control and Prevention guidelines on social distancing, contractors reported purchasing personal protective equipment, increasing cleaning at facilities, and buying additional equipment to support teleworking. Contractors also reported that they adjusted their internal policies, such as increasing telework availability, allowing flexible employee schedules, implementing shift work, and enhancing leave share programs. To keep employees working, 11 out of the 15 contractors in our review reported moving employees to different contracts or projects.

Some large prime contractors in our review also took steps to lessen the effect of COVID-19 disruptions on their supply chain. In their financial statements, they reported using increased progress payment rates from the government to accelerate payments to subcontractors so the industrial base could maintain its financial health and liquidity. Further, some of these contractors' representatives told us that accelerating payments to critical suppliers and subcontractors was helpful in minimizing the effect of COVID-19.

Contractor representatives told us that after taking steps to keep employees working, there was still a need to provide paid leave to some employees.[29] However, the proportion of employees and contracts for which each contractor requested paid leave reimbursement was usually low compared to the contractor's overall workforce and contracting base. For example, as of February 2021, 14 of the 15 contractors in our review reported seeking reimbursement on a subset, rather than all, of their federal contracts. Representatives of one contractor told us that they sought section 3610 reimbursement on only 1 percent of their contracts. Representatives of another contractor stated that as of January 2021, they had three employees for whom they were currently requesting reimbursement under section 3610, representing less than 1 percent of their workforce.

---

[29] Some contractors we spoke with told us they also incurred paid leave costs or used section 3610 in their work with the Intelligence Community.

Conclusion

In the face of the pandemic, provisions to keep the government and its contractor support in a ready state—such as section 3610—could help accelerate recovery. Agencies understandably prioritized quick implementation of section 3610 over a more deliberative process given the urgency of responding to the pandemic. For a number of reasons, agencies' use and implementation of section 3610 authority, and contractors' experiences, varied. Once the COVID-19 pandemic is over, there will be an opportunity for the federal government—with the coordination of OMB's OFPP—to collect and share lessons learned from agencies' implementation of section 3610. Doing so could enhance how agencies implement paid leave reimbursement provisions should they be enacted in response to future emergencies.

Recommendation for Executive Action

The Director of OMB should, upon conclusion of the COVID-19 national emergency, ensure that OFPP collects and shares lessons learned from federal agencies' implementation of COVID-19 paid leave reimbursement, including those related to data tracking and reporting. (Recommendation 1)

Agency Comments

We provided a draft of this report to DHS, DOD, DOE, NASA and OMB for review and comment. DHS and NASA had no comments on the draft report. DOD and DOE provided technical comments, which we incorporated as appropriate. OMB concurred with the recommendation. In an email response, OMB noted that OFPP seeks to promote interagency collaboration and sharing of information and lessons learned. OMB further noted that after the enactment of section 3610, OFPP convened senior procurement executives and FAR Council members on several occasions to discuss OFPP's guiding principles and to provide a forum for agencies to explain their approaches and share perspectives on implementation. In addition, OFPP posted agencies' public guidance documents on a government-wide coronavirus acquisition-related website and posted internal information in an OMB system used to facilitate collaboration. OFPP agreed to collect and share individual agencies' lessons learned more broadly with the community to promote knowledge management.

We are sending copies of this report to the appropriate congressional addressees; the Secretaries of Defense, Energy, and Homeland Security; the Administrator of NASA; and the Acting Director of OMB. In addition, the report will be made available at no charge on the GAO website at https://www.gao.gov.

If you or your staff have any questions concerning this report, please contact me at (202) 512-4841. Contact points for our offices of Congressional Relations and Public Affairs may be found on the last page of this report. Staff members making key contributions to this report are listed in appendix II.

Timothy J. DiNapoli
Director, Contracting and National Security Acquisitions

List of Addressees

The Honorable Patrick Leahy
Chairman

The Honorable Richard Shelby
Vice Chairman
Committee on Appropriations
United States Senate

The Honorable Ron Wyden
Chairman

The Honorable Mike Crapo
Ranking Member
Committee on Finance
United States Senate

The Honorable Patty Murray
Chair

The Honorable Richard Burr
Ranking Member
Committee on Health, Education, Labor, and Pensions
United States Senate

The Honorable Gary C. Peters
Chair

The Honorable Rob Portman
Ranking Member

Committee on Homeland Security
and Governmental Affairs
United States Senate

The Honorable Rosa L. DeLauro
Chairwoman

The Honorable Kay Granger
Ranking Member
Committee on Appropriations
House of Representatives

The Honorable Robert C. "Bobby" Scott
Chairman

The Honorable Virginia Foxx
Ranking Member
Committee on Education and Labor
House of Representatives

The Honorable Frank Pallone, Jr.
Chairman

The Honorable Cathy McMorris Rodgers
Republican Leader
Committee on Energy and Commerce
House of Representatives

The Honorable Bennie G. Thompson
Chairman
House of Representatives

The Honorable John Katko
Ranking Member
Committee on Homeland Security
House of Representatives

The Honorable Carolyn B. Maloney
Chairwoman
The Honorable James Comer
Ranking Member
Committee on Oversight and Reform
House of Representatives

The Honorable Eddie Bernice Johnson
Chairwoman
Committee on Science, Space, and Technology
House of Representatives

The Honorable Richard E. Neal
Chairman

The Honorable Kevin Brady
Republican Leader
Committee on Ways and Means
House of Representatives

The Honorable Donald S. Beyer, Jr.
Chairman
Subcommittee on Space and Aeronautics Committee on Science, Space, and Technology

Appendix I: Objectives, Scope, and Methodology

This report (1) examines how selected federal agencies have used section 3610 authority and (2) presents selected contractors' perspectives on Coronavirus Disease 2019 (COVID-19) paid leave reimbursement.

To examine how selected federal agencies have used section 3610 authority, we identified the seven federal agencies with contract obligations greater than $10 billion in fiscal year 2019—the most recent full year for which data were available at the time of our analysis. We reviewed these agencies' use of section 3610 authority as of July 20, 2020, as reported to the Federal Procurement Data System (FPDS), and selected the three agencies with reported use. These three agencies were the Department of Defense (DOD), Department of Energy (DOE), and the National Aeronautics and Space Administration (NASA). As a point of comparison, we also selected one agency—the Department of Homeland Security (DHS)—that had not reported use of section 3610 authority as of July 20, 2020.[1] For these four agencies, we gathered and analyzed guidance regarding section 3610 and data on its use either collected by agencies or reported to FPDS from January 31, 2020, through March 31, 2021; and interviewed or received written responses from cognizant agency officials.[2] We also interviewed officials from the Office of Management and Budget's (OMB) Office of Federal Procurement Policy (OFPP) regarding the extent of this agency's plans to collect and share lessons learned from federal agencies' implementation of section 3610, due to this agency's role in coordinating government- wide contracting policy. To assess the reliability of data from agencies and FPDS, we reviewed related documentation such as data validation rules and interviewed knowledgeable agency officials. We determined the data were sufficiently reliable for the purposes of describing the extent to which selected agencies reported use of

---

[1] In addition, the scope of this engagement does not include use of section 3610 within the Intelligence Community. We coordinated with the Office of Inspector General of the National Reconnaissance Office, which completed an evaluation of that agency's implementation of section 3610 in January 2021. National Reconnaissance Office, Office of Inspector General, *Evaluation of the National Reconnaissance Office's Implementation of Section 3610 Authorized by the Coronavirus Aid, Relief, and Economic Security Act*, Project Number 2020-004 S (Chantilly, VA: Jan. 4, 2021).

[2] According to the General Services Administration, FPDS is the federal government's authoritative source for contract data. Contracts whose estimated value is $10,000 or more are reported to FPDS, as well as every modification to those contracts, regardlessof dollar value. On October 17, 2020, the FPDS reports module was retired and the https://SAM.gov Data Bank is now the only place to create and run both standard and ad hoc reports on federal contract data.

section 3610 authority. To identify selected contractors' perspectives on COVID-19 paid leave reimbursement, we selected a non-generalizable sample of 15 prime contractors that, according to agency data, have received or requested section 3610 reimbursements from one or more agencies in this review. These contractors reflected a range of company sizes, ownership structures, and product and service offerings. We selected the following 15 contractors:

- Afognak Native Corporation
- ASRC Federal Holding Company
- The Boeing Company
- Booz Allen Hamilton Holding Corporation
- Constellis
- Fluor Corporation
- General Dynamics Corporation
- Jacobs Engineering Group Inc.
- Leidos Holdings, Inc.
- Lockheed Martin Corporation
- Melwood Horticultural Training Center, Inc.
- Northrop Grumman Corporation
- Raytheon Technologies Corporation
- S&K Technologies, Inc.
- Science and Technology Corporation

We conducted semi-structured interviews of cognizant contractor representatives about their experiences seeking reimbursement from different agencies and reviewed available company financial information. We also interviewed representatives from the following industry associations about contractors' experiences seeking reimbursement from different agencies, and about why some contractors have not requested reimbursements:

- Aerospace Industries Association
- Coalition for Government Procurement
- National Defense Industrial Association
- Professional Services Council
- Shipbuilders Council of America

Additionally, we selected four contractors that we identified as having not yet requested section 3610 reimbursements from agencies in our review at the time of selection. For each of the four agencies in our review, we identified the three contractors with the most contract obligations in fiscal year 2020, as reported to FPDS, that did not appear in agencies' lists of contractors that had received or requested section 3610 reimbursements, and that FPDS showed as having not received contract obligations indicating use of section 3610 authority. We then selected one of the three contractors from each agency to reflect a range of company sizes, ownership structures, and product and service offerings. Based on this analysis, we interviewed or received written responses from cognizant representatives from the following four contractors:

- Association of Universities for Research in Astronomy
- Huntington Ingalls Industries, Inc.
- The GEO Group, Inc.
- Project Enhancement Corporation

We conducted this performance audit from October 2020 to July 2021 in accordance with generally accepted government auditing standards.

Those standards require that we plan and perform the audit to obtain sufficient, appropriate evidence to provide a reasonable basis for our findings and conclusions based on our audit objectives. We believe that the evidence obtained provides a reasonable basis for our findings and conclusions based on our audit objectives.

Appendix II: Staff Acknowledgments

In addition to the contact named above, Tatiana Winger (Assistant Director), Sarah Amer, Hilary Benedict, Robert Bullock (Analyst-in- Charge), Laura Greifner, Julia Kennon, Natalie Logan, Miranda Riemer, Zamir Ruli, Rachel Stoiko, Roxanna Sun, and Carmen Yeung made key contributions to this report.

Chapter 4

COVID-19 Contracting: Indian Health Service Used Flexibilities to Meet Increased Medical Supply Needs*

United States Government Accountability Office

Abbreviations

AI/AN	American Indian and Alaska Native
COVID-19	Coronavirus Disease 2019
DHS	Department of Homeland Security
DOD	Department of Defense
FAR	Federal Acquisition Regulation
FPDS	Federal Procurement Data System
GSA	General Services Administration
HHS	Department of Health and Human Services
IHS	Indian Health Service
NSSC	National Supply Service Center
PPV	pharmaceutical prime vendor
U.S.C.	U.S. Code
WHO	World Health Organization

* This is an edited, reformatted and augmented version of the United States Government Accountability Office Report to Congressional Addressees, Publication No. GAO-22-104745, dated October 2021.

In: COVID-19 Contracting
Editor: Eric Neudorf
ISBN: 978-1-68507-710-5

Why This Matters

The Indian Health Service (IHS) serves over 2 million American Indians and Alaska Natives. These groups have been disproportionately vulnerable to negative outcomes from COVID-19. During emergencies, federal contracting staff face pressure to work quickly to meet increased needs. We examined some of IHS's COVID- related contracts to see how the agency's efforts fared.

Key Takeaways

Despite facing challenges, including unprecedented demand for medical supplies, IHS was able to acquire needed products from a variety of vendors. IHS contract obligations for products, excluding prescription drugs, increased substantially during COVID-19 to address emergent needs for additional personal protective equipment, lab supplies, and more. Using emergency contracting flexibilities available under federal regulation, HIS

- bought personal protective equipment and other medical products in bulk
- awarded contracts noncompetitively
- used streamlined procedures for higher dollar contracts to obtain medical supplies faster

However, we found that IHS contracting officers did not notice that some COVID-related supplies were delivered late. Officials attributed this oversight to the spike in volume as well as the urgency of procurements during a pandemic.

Contracting officers are responsible for ensuring the terms of a contract are met—under normal circumstances and in emergency acquisitions. IHS officials told us that they began taking intermediate steps to improve tracking of products during 2020; the agency is currently obtaining new software to improve contractor oversight.

How GAO Did This Study

We analyzed relevant federal procurement data through June 30, 2021. We also reviewed four contracts— covering about 1/4 of obligations in IHS's largest product category (medical and surgical instruments, equipment, and supplies). We also interviewed IHS contracting officials.

IHS Contract Obligations Increased Substantially Due to COVID-19

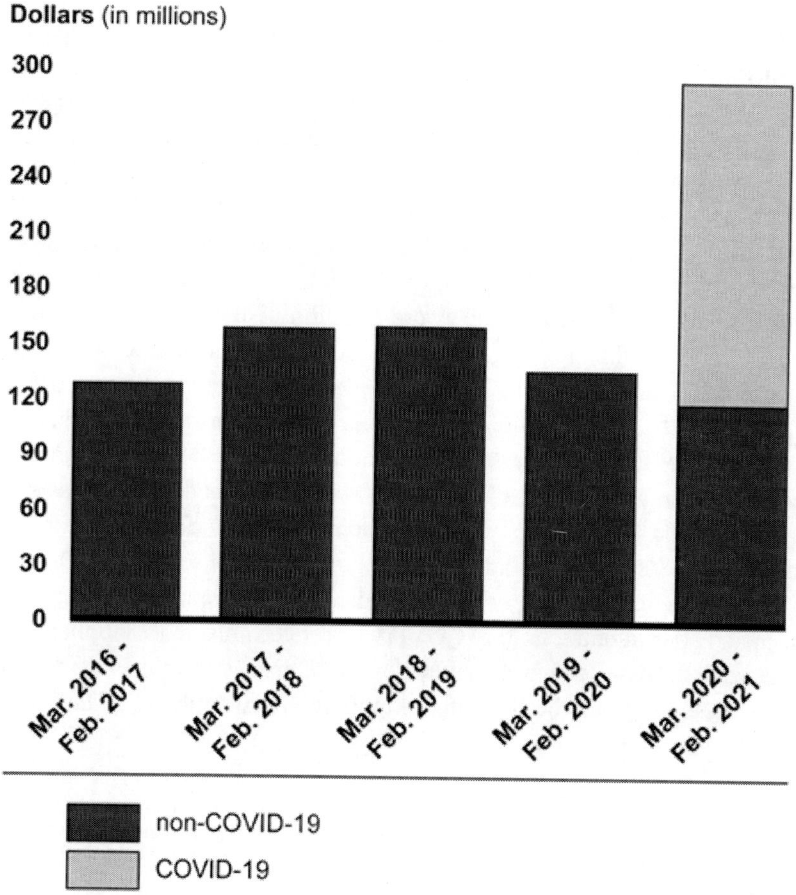

Source: GAO analysis of Federal Procurement Data System data. | GAO-22-104745.

October 14, 2021
Congressional Addressees

Coronavirus Disease 2019 (COVID-19) has put the U.S. health care system, including the Indian Health Service (IHS), under severe strain, affecting the federal government's ability to buy and maintain critical medical supplies to treat patients and protect health care workers. IHS provides comprehensive health services for American Indians and Alaska Natives (AI/AN)—a population that has long experienced lower life expectancy and health disparities compared to other Americans.

Our prior work found that contracts play a key role in federal emergency response efforts, and that contracting during an emergency can present a unique set of challenges as officials can face significant pressure to provide critical goods and services as expeditiously and efficiently as possible.[1]

You requested that we review IHS's contracting efforts for COVID-19 medical supplies. This report examines (1) the key characteristics of IHS's contract obligations for COVID-19-related products, including medical supplies, and (2) the contracting approaches IHS used to buy medical supplies and any challenges it faced in the award and administration of those contracts.

To conduct this review, we analyzed data available in the Federal Procurement Data System (FPDS) as of June 30, 2021 to identify the IHS area offices with the most contract obligations and obtain detailed information about those contracts.[2] We assessed the reliability of FPDS data by reviewing existing information about the FPDS system and the data it collects, and determined the FPDS data were sufficiently reliable for the purposes of describing IHS's reported contract obligations in response to COVID-19.

Based on those data, we then selected and reviewed the five largest completed IHS contracts for COVID-19-related medical supplies as of January 25, 2021, when we began this review. During our review, we excluded one of these contracts because it was potentially the subject of an ongoing

---

[1] GAO, Disaster Contracting: FEMA Continues to Face Challenges with Its Use of Contracts to Support Response and Recovery, GAO-19-518T (Washington, D.C.: May 9, 2019); 2017 Disaster Contracting: Actions Needed to Improve the Use of Post-Disaster Contracts to Support Response and Recovery, GAO-19-281 (Washington, D.C.: Apr. 24, 2019); 2017 Disaster Contracting: Action Needed to Better Ensure More Effective Use and Management of Advance Contracts, GAO-19-93 (Washington, D.C.: Dec. 6, 2018).

[2] For the purposes of this report, "contract obligations" means obligations on contracts that are subject to the Federal Acquisition Regulation, and does not include, for example, grants, cooperative agreements, loans, other transactions for research, real property leases, or requisitions from federal stock.

Office of Inspector General investigation.[3] We also interviewed the cognizant contracting officers for these contracts as well as officials at IHS headquarters and the IHS National Supply Service Center (NSSC), which manages a large portion of IHS's COVID-19 contracts. Finally, we reviewed IHS's procurement policies and relevant portions of the Federal Acquisition Regulation (FAR). Further details about the scope and methodology for this work can be found in appendix I.

We conducted this performance audit from January 2021 to October 2021 in accordance with generally accepted government auditing standards.

Those standards require that we plan and perform the audit to obtain sufficient, appropriate evidence to provide a reasonable basis for our findings and conclusions based on our audit objectives. We believe that the evidence obtained provides a reasonable basis for our findings and conclusions based on our audit objectives.

Background

IHS, an agency within the Department of Health and Human Services (HHS), provides health care for over 2 million AI/AN people who are members or descendants of federally recognized tribes.[4] We previously reported that AI/AN people tend to experience health disparities when compared to other Americans.[5] As of October 2019, AI/AN people had a life expectancy that was 5.5 years less than all other races or ethnicities in the U.S. and died at higher rates than other Americans from many preventable causes, including diabetes mellitus and chronic lower respiratory diseases. AI/AN individuals with these health conditions are at greater risk of developing serious complications from COVID-19.[6]

IHS provides services directly through a network of hospitals, clinics, and health stations it operates, and it funds services provided at tribally operated

---

[3] We refer to the four remaining contracts we reviewed as Contracts A, B, C, and D.

[4] Federally recognized tribes have a government-to-government relationship with the U.S. and are eligible to receive certain protections, services, and benefits by virtue of their status as Indian tribes. The Secretary of the Interior publishes a list of all tribal entities that the Secretary recognizes as Indian tribes annually in the Federal Register. As of January 29, 2021 there were 574 federally recognized tribes. See 86 Fed. Reg. 7554 (Jan. 29, 2021).

[5] GAO, *COVID-19: Opportunities to Improve Federal Response and Recovery Efforts*, GAO-20-625 (Washington, D.C.: June 25, 2020).

[6] GAO-20-625.

facilities.[7] IHS also provides funding to nonprofit, urban Indian organizations through the Urban Indian Health program to provide health care services to AI/AN people living in urban areas.

IHS administers services through a system of 12 area offices and 170 IHS and tribally operated service units. IHS's 12 area offices serve different geographic regions within the U.S., as shown in figure 1. Each area has its own contracting office, which is responsible for awarding and administering contracts in that area.

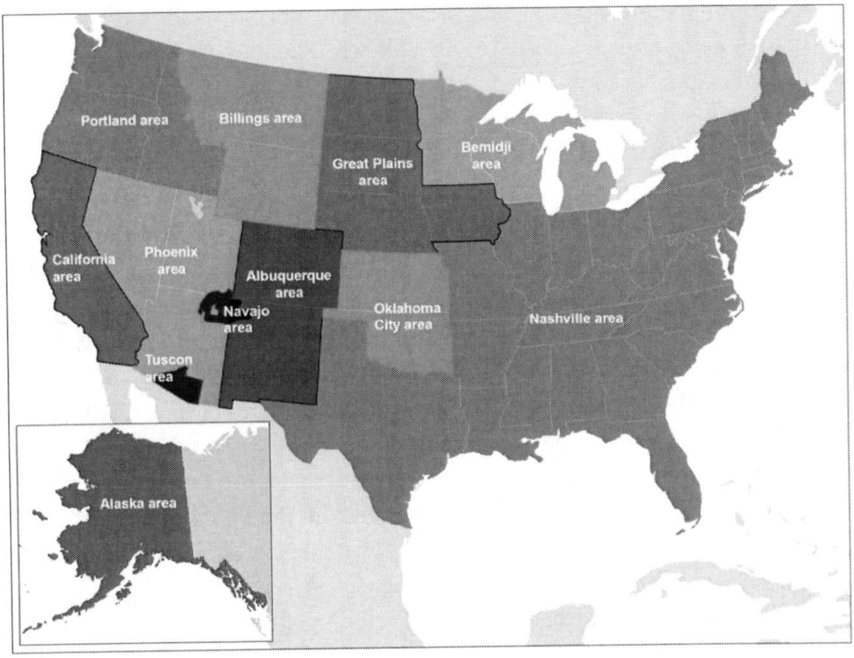

Source: Indian Health Service. | GAO-22-104745.

Figure 1. Map of Indian Health Service Area Offices.

Within the Oklahoma City area office, IHS has the NSSC, which coordinates large national contracts. NSSC is a focus of our review because it managed a large portion of IHS's contracting for COVID-19- related products, including medical supplies.

---

[7] See 25 U.S.C. § 1653.

COVID-19 Timeline of Events

- December 2019 – A new strain of coronavirus emerged and quickly spread around the globe.
- March 11, 2020 – The World Health Organization declared the outbreak of COVID-19 a pandemic.
- March 13, 2020 – The President of the U.S. declared a national emergency, pursuant to the National Emergencies Act and under section 501(b) of the Robert T. Stafford Disaster Relief and Emergency Assistance Act (Stafford Act).
- As of July 24, 2021, IHS reported 204,197 confirmed COVID-19 cases among those receiving care at IHS facilities.

Federal Regulations and Agency-specific Acquisition Guidance

The FAR establishes uniform policies and procedures for acquisition by all executive agencies, including requirements for planning and competition for awarding contracts. Although agencies generally must use full and open competition when awarding contracts, the FAR provides exceptions, such as when an agency's need for supplies or services is of such "unusual and compelling urgency" that the government would suffer serious harm unless it is permitted to limit the sources from which it solicits the supplies or services. In addition, the FAR states that it is the policy of the government to provide maximum practicable opportunities in acquisitions to small businesses.

IHS also follows HHS's acquisition regulation that supplements the FAR. In addition, Part 5, Chapter 5 of the Indian Health Manual identifies, explains, and clarifies IHS's policies and procedures for acquisition management.

IHS Has Obligated Millions of Dollars on New Contracts for COVID-19-Related Products

IHS obligations for medical supplies increased substantially after the COVID-19 national emergency declaration, primarily through new, noncompetitive contracts used to obtain a variety of critical products.[8] The agency's contract

[8] For purposes of this report, "noncompetitive contracts" refers to contracts and orders identified with certain codes in FPDS, as explained in detail in appendix I of this report. Even for

obligations for products in response to the pandemic totaled more than $206 million as of June 30, 2021. Contract obligations peaked in April 2020 and again in January 2021.

According to FPDS data, the first peak included substantial purchases of masks and gloves, and the second peak was primarily driven by an agency-wide contract for lab analyzers, test kits, and reagents to test COVID-19 samples. Figure 2 illustrates IHS contract obligations by month for COVID-19-related products since the start of the pandemic.

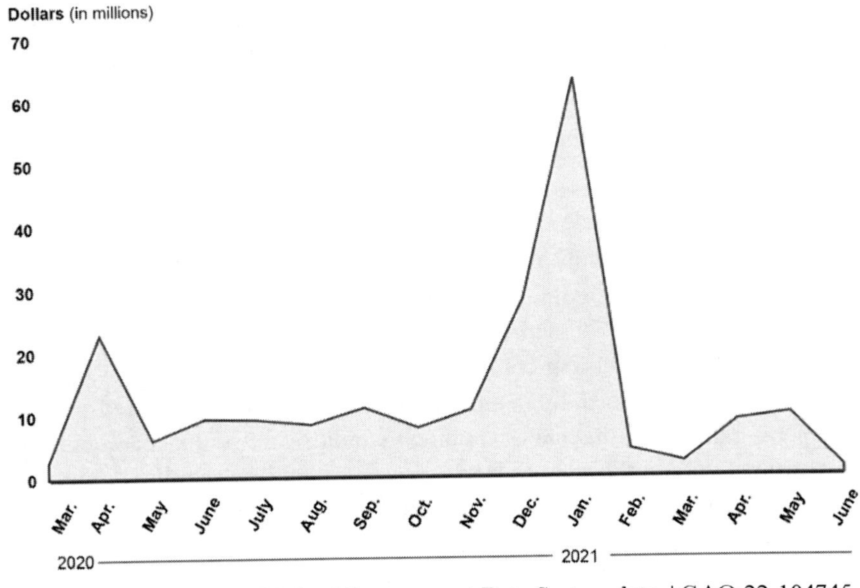

Source: GAO analysis of Federal Procurement Data System data. | GAO-22-104745.

Figure 2. Timeline of Indian Health Service Contract Obligations for COVID-19-Related Products by Month, as of June 30, 2021.

Overall IHS obligations for non-pharmaceutical products (such as gloves, masks, and gowns) increased substantially after the COVID-19 national emergency declaration.[9] For example, IHS obligated $293 million for non-

contracts and orders identified with these codes, agencies may have solicited more than one source.

[9] For purposes of Figure 3, we removed obligations for the pharmacy prime vendor (PPV) program from our calculations. IHS officials said that prior to August 2019, FPDS data included all obligations for the PPV program. IHS officials added that since August 2019, IHS has not reported PPV obligations for tribally-operated facilities in FPDS to ensure accurate reporting of IHS-specific obligations in FPDS.

pharmaceutical products in the first 12 months of the national emergency, compared to $136 million during the 12-month period before the March 2020 declaration (see figure 3).

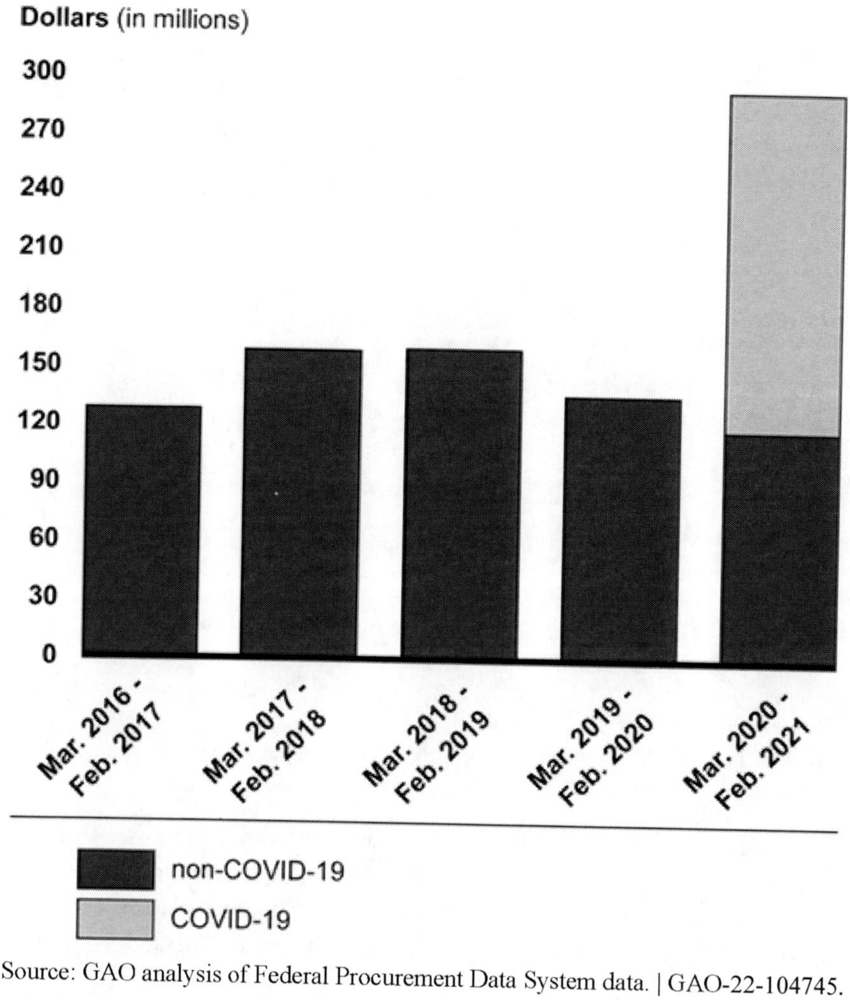

Source: GAO analysis of Federal Procurement Data System data. | GAO-22-104745.

Figure 3. Indian Health Service Contract Obligations on Non-Pharmaceutical Products, March 2016 through February 2021.

IHS procured a variety of critical products in response to the pandemic. The top five product types accounted for 90 percent of total obligations for COVID-19-related products. For example, medical and surgical instruments, equipment, and supplies accounted for nearly $91 million, or 44 percent, of obligations for COVID-19-related products. Figure 4 shows the top five products by contract obligations.

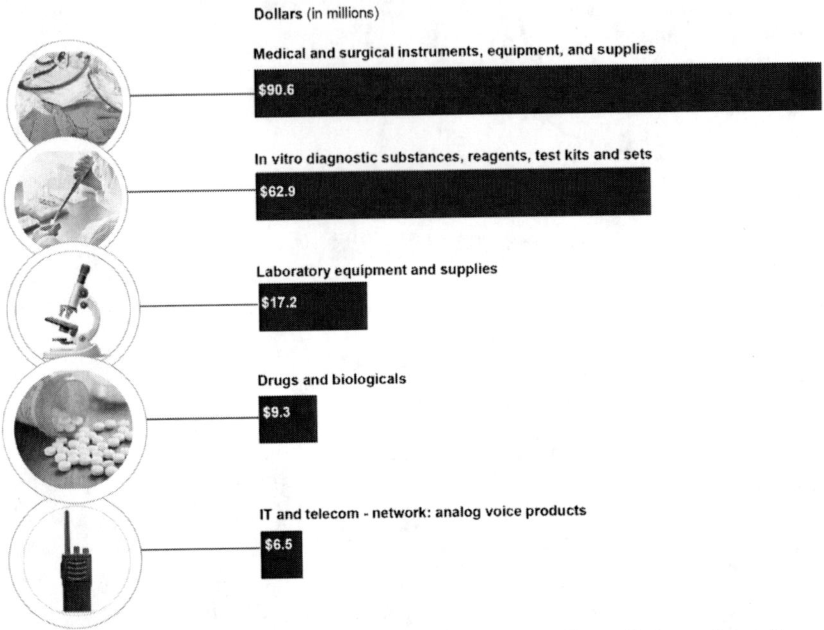

Source: (data) GAO Analysis of Federal Procurement Data System data; (images) Sherry Young, tilialucida, belokrylowa, JJava, Kontur-vid, stock.adobe.com. | GAO-22-104745.

Figure 4. Top Five Products Procured in Response to COVID-19 by Indian Health Service, as of June 30, 2021.

Most of IHS's COVID-19-related contract obligations reported in FPDS, about $169 million, were for new contracts, compared with about $37 million in obligations on pre-existing contracts.[10] Almost three-quarters of IHS's COVID-19 obligations for products were on contracts identified as awarded noncompetitively, as shown in figure 5.

[10] New contract obligations include obligations on new definitive contracts (as reported in FPDS), purchase orders, indefinite delivery vehicles, and blanket purchase agreements awarded or established after March 17, 2020—the date of the first IHS contract obligations in response to COVID-19—and all associated orders, calls, and modifications to these awards. Preexisting contract obligations include obligations on orders, calls, and modifications to definitive contracts, purchase orders, indefinite delivery vehicles, and blanket purchase agreements awarded or established prior to March 17, 2020.

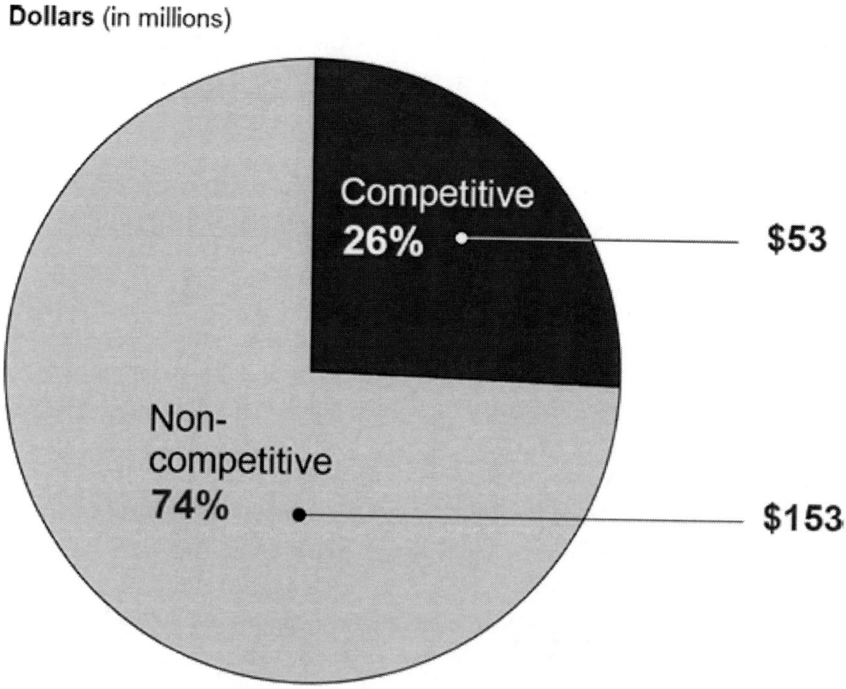

Source: GAO analysis of Federal Procurement Data System data. | GAO-22-104745.
Note: For purposes of this report, noncompetitive contracts refers to contracts and orders identified with certain codes in the Federal Procurement Data System, as explained in detail in appendix I of this report. Even for contracts and orders identified with these codes, agencies may have solicited more than one source.

Figure 5. Competitive Versus Noncompetitive Indian Health Service Contracts for COVID-19-Related Products, as of June 30, 2021.

Most of the contracts awarded noncompetitively (74 percent) cited the unusual and compelling urgency exception to full and open competition.[11]

As with the federal government overall, competition rates for IHS contracts during the pandemic were much lower than normal due to the national emergency. From fiscal years 2015 through 2019, IHS contracts were awarded noncompetitively, on average, almost 19 percent of the time, compared to 74 percent during the pandemic.

[11] Our methodology for identifying noncompetitive contracts is explained in detail in appendix I of this report. Even for contracts identified as noncompetitive, agencies may have solicited more than one source.

In addition, about 43 percent of IHS's COVID-19 contract obligations were for products provided by small businesses.

IHS Adapted Its Contracting Approach to Address COVID-19 Challenges, but Was Unaware of Some Delivery Delays

IHS used available emergency contracting flexibilities and increased bulk purchases to meet its COVID-19 medical supply needs. However, contracting officials experienced challenges due to the increased volume and urgency of procurements and were unaware that vendors delivered some supplies late.

IHS Used Contracting Flexibilities and Increased Bulk Purchases to Meet Its COVID-19 Medical Supply Needs

IHS responded to COVID-19-related medical supply challenges by using acquisition flexibilities available in the FAR for emergency acquisitions to streamline its procurement of goods and services, including the following:

- *Unusual and compelling urgency* - Provides an exception to the general requirement for full and open competition when an agency's need for supplies or services is of such "unusual and compelling urgency" that the government would suffer serious harm unless it is permitted to limit the sources from which it solicits the supplies of goods or services.[12]
- *Increased simplified acquisition threshold* – Increases the threshold for using simplified acquisition procedures from $250,000 to $800,000 for acquisitions in the U.S. to support a response to an emergency or major disaster declared under the Robert T. Stafford Disaster Relief and Emergency Assistance Act.[13] For purchases at or below the simplified acquisition threshold, agencies may use

[12] On March 21, 2020, the HHS senior procurement executive issued a class justification and approval that generally authorized HHS contracting offices to award contracts under the unusual and compelling urgency exception to full and open competition for COVID-19-related procurements.

[13] At the outset of the period covered by our review, the simplified acquisition threshold for acquisitions in the U.S. to support a response to an emergency or major disaster was $750,000. Effective October 1, 2020, the FAR was amended to increase this threshold to $800,000. 85 Fed. Reg. 62,485, 62,487 (Oct. 2, 2020).

streamlined procurement procedures, called “simplified acquisition procedures.”

- *Increased threshold for simplified procedures for commercial items* – Increases the threshold for using simplified acquisition procedures for commercial items from $7.5 million to $15 million for purchases to support a response to an emergency or major disaster declared under the Robert T. Stafford Disaster Relief and Emergency Assistance Act.[14]

Further, on March 21, 2020, HHS’s senior procurement executive granted a waiver of the requirement for detailed, formal acquisition plans for all COVID-19-related acquisitions above the simplified acquisition threshold, allowing HHS contracting activities to use HHS’s Streamlined Acquisition Plan template instead.[15]

Additionally, on April 2, 2020, the head of contracting activity for the Navajo Area Indian Health Service authorized the acquisition of personal protective equipment for the COVID-19 response without regard to restrictions in the Buy American Act or the Trade Agreements Act, based on exceptions to those restrictions. The Buy American Act establishes a preference that only domestic end products be acquired for public use.

The act, however, permits federal agencies to procure foreign products under certain exceptions, such as where domestic products are not reasonably available in sufficient quantities of a satisfactory quality.[16] The Trade Agreements Act, as implemented by the FAR, requires the acquisition of only U.S.-made or designated country end products or U.S. or designated country

[14] At the outset of the period covered by our review, these thresholds, as implemented in the FAR, were $7 million and $13 million, respectively. Effective October 1, 2020, the FAR was amended to increase these thresholds to $7.5 million and $15 million, respectively. 85 Fed. Reg. 62,485, 62,488 (Oct. 2, 2020).

[15] In general, acquisition plans detail milestones at which decisions should be made for an acquisition as well as all the technical, business, management, and other significant considerations that will control the acquisition. See FAR § 7.105. The HHS Acquisition Regulation references the content requirements for a written acquisition plan in the FAR and requires a written acquisition plan for all acquisitions above the simplified acquisition threshold.

[16] 41 U.S.C. § 8302; FAR § 25.101, 25.102, 25.103. The head of contracting activity for the Navajo Area Indian Health Service cited this exception in the authorization for the acquisition of COVID-19-related personal protective equipment without Buy American Act restrictions.

services, unless offers for such products or services are insufficient for the requirements.[17]

Figure 6 illustrates key events in IHS's procurement response to the COVID-19 pandemic, including the implementation of contracting flexibilities and award dates for the four selected contracts in our review.

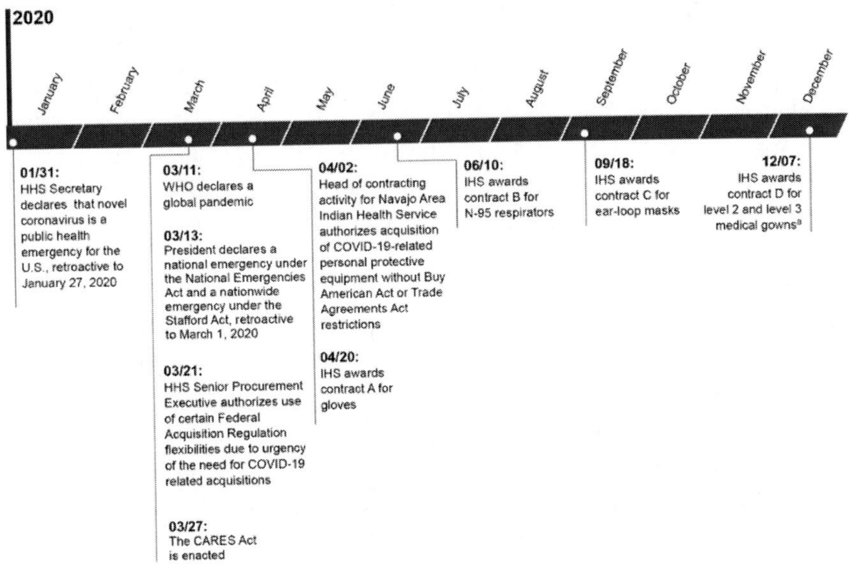

IHS	Indian Health Service
HHS	Department of Health and Human Services
WHO	World Health Organization

Source: GAO analysis of HIS documentation and GAO-20-625. | GAO-22-104745.

Note: We refer to the four selected Indian Health Service contracts as Contracts A, B, C, and D.

[a] According to the Food and Drug Administration, level 2 gowns offer barrier protection for low risk settings, whereas level 3 gowns offer barrier protection for moderate risk setting s.

Figure 6. COVID-19-Related Events and Award Dates for Four Selected Indian Health Service (IHS) Contracts.

---

[17] 19 U.S.C. § 2512(a); FAR § 25.403(c). In the authorization for the acquisition of COVID- 19-related personal protective equipment without Trade Agreements Act restrictions, the head of contracting activity for the Navajo Area Indian Health Service cited an exception for acquisitions that do not use full and open competition.

Our review of the four large IHS medical supply contracts found that three of those contracts used at least one of the acquisition flexibilities previously discussed (see table 1). Use of these flexibilities allowed IHS to award these contracts soon after identifying a vendor that could meet its needs.

Table 1. Acquisition Flexibilities Used for Selected Contracts

	Acquisition Flexibility				
Contract	Class Justification & Approval for noncompetitive award based on urgency	Increased Simplified Acquisition Threshold	Increased Commercia l Items Threshold	Streamlined Acquisition Plan	Waived Buy American Act and Trade Agreement Act Restrictions
Contract A (gloves)	—	—	—	✓	—
Contract B (N-95 respirators)	—	—	—	—	—
Contract C (ear-loop masks)	—	—	—	✓	—
Contract D (level 2 and level 3 medical gowns)	✓	—	✓	✓	—

Source: GAO Analysis of Indian Health Service contract files and Federal Procurement Data System data. | GAO-22-104745.

Note: "—" indicates the flexibility was not applicable to the procurement or the contract file did not reflect that IHS used the flexibility.

"√" indicates the contract file reflected that IHS used the acquisition flexibility.

IHS officials told us that awarding contracts quickly was important because the medical supply market was volatile, and the availability of items could rapidly change. In addition, some existing vendors were unable to deliver medical supplies at the time.

For example, IHS relied on an existing agreement for purchasing gowns prior to the pandemic, but the vendor was unable to deliver needed quantities once the COVID-19 pandemic began. As a result, IHS had to identify another vendor for gowns, which led to Contract D. Likewise, IHS terminated Contract B for the government's convenience after the vendor was unable to obtain the N-95 respirators from the manufacturer within the time frame specified in the contract.

IHS also responded to COVID-19 challenges by increasing bulk purchases of medical products by NSSC. While NSSC's overall mission has remained unchanged during the COVID-19 emergency, according to IHS officials, the volume of supplies procured by NSSC and the number of customers served have increased, and the urgency of the procurements has escalated.

Responding to these increased demands, IHS provided $398 million in funding to NSSC to coordinate and manage the purchase and distribution of COVID-19-related medical products nationwide to IHS and tribal medical facilities and urban medical centers.[18] NSSC provided these supplies at no cost to the facilities and centers. Under normal circumstances, NSSC recovers costs by charging reimbursement fees to the medical facilities.

NSSC determined IHS's COVID-19 medical supply needs by working with IHS's 12 area offices to calculate cumulative medical supply usage rates. The Oklahoma City Area accounted for $135.1 million of the $206 million obligated (see figure 7).

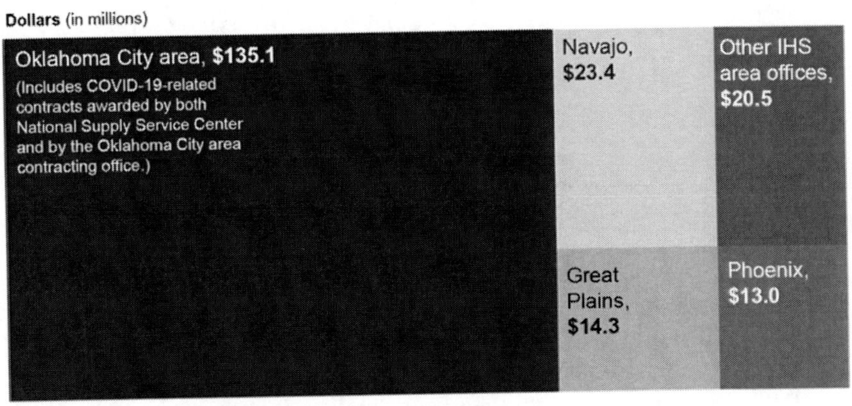

Source: GAO analysis of Federal Procurement Data Syste data. | GAO-22-104745.

Figure 7. Contract Obligations for Products in Response to COVID-19 by Indian Health Service (IHS) Area Office, as of June 30, 2021.

---

[18] IHS provided $398 million to NSSC to procure personal protective equipment and other medical supplies for IHS, tribal, and urban medical facilities at no cost to the facilities. Of this, $10 million was included in an appropriation to IHS under the CARES Act. IHS officials report that the remaining $388 million came primarily from HHS's Public Health and Social Services Emergency Fund to prevent, prepare for, and respond to coronavirus. According to IHS officials, some of these funds are available through fiscal year 2024, and some are available until expended.

Contracting Officials Experienced COVID-19 Challenges and Were Unaware of Late Deliveries

IHS officials stated that their greatest challenge was dealing with the increased volume of supplies and urgency of procurements during the COVID-19 emergency and that this contributed to the lack of awareness that vendors delivered some products late.[19] IHS officials stated that, as a whole, however, the agency considered these acquisitions successful because they were able to acquire the needed supplies during a national emergency.

We found that deliveries for masks and gowns under contracts C and D were late, according to the terms of the contracts. During initial interviews about the contracts under review, IHS officials told us that the vendors for each of the four contracts we reviewed, except for the vendor whose contract was terminated, delivered all supplies on time. However, we determined that the vendor for contracts C and D delivered some quantities late on both contracts. For example, our analysis found that, under the contract for level 2 and level 3 gowns, the vendor delivered about 20 percent of the level 2 gowns and about 35 percent of the level 3 gowns up to 1 month late. Under the contract for ear-loop masks, the vendor delivered about 6 percent of masks up to 10 days late. For both contracts, the contracting officer acknowledged that they were unaware the supplies were delivered late until we identified the discrepancy.

The Indian Health Manual states that the key to effective contract administration is constantly monitoring contractor performance. The manual also states that, after contract award, a project officer is responsible for tracking contract progress and for advising the contracting officer, in writing, of contractor performance, including monitoring the delivery of acceptable contractor supplies or services according to contract terms and conditions.

IHS officials stated that warehouse staff at NSSC's distribution warehouse generate reports documenting delivery and acceptance once products are successfully delivered. These reports—known as receiving reports—are provided to the contracting officer via intra-office mail.

---

[19] GAO reviewed four NSSC contract files. No deliveries were made under Contract B, and it was terminated for convenience by the government. Contract A was fulfilled on time. Contracts C and D both involved late deliveries. The FAR provides that contracting officers are responsible for ensuring performance of all necessary actions for effective contracting, ensuring compliance with the terms of the contract, and safeguarding the interests of the U.S. in its contractual relationships. FAR § 1.602-2.

Officials added that these receiving reports should be included in the contract file. Although receiving reports were prepared and, according to NSSC officials, a hard copy of each report was delivered to the contracting officer, contracting officials did not realize that supplies ordered under contracts C and D were not delivered according to the schedule terms identified in the contracts.

IHS contracting officials stated that during the COVID-19 emergency, the workload of the contracting and NSSC warehouse staff increased significantly because of the volume of supplies being procured and delivered. IHS officials stated that, under normal circumstances, either the contracting or NSSC warehouse staff would have noticed if products were not yet received or delivered late. In these instances, the contracting officer would have contacted the vendor and discussed possible corrective actions.

NSSC officials stated that they recognized in 2020 the need for improvements in their ability to track supplies during the COVID-19 emergency. As a result, NSSC began implementing procedural changes, including maintaining daily logs of all supplies delivered. These actions are still underway and have not been fully implemented. In addition, NSSC officials stated that they recently procured new software that will enable real-time tracking of deliveries and improved communication between warehouse and contracting staff. NSSC is currently developing internal guidance for the use of this software and plans to have the software fully deployed to track all supply procurements within NSSC by October 2021.

Agency Comments

We provided a draft of this report to the Department of Health and Human Services for review and comment. The agency provided technical comments which we incorporated as appropriate.

We are also sending copies of this report to the appropriate congressional committees and offices. In addition, the report will be made available at no charge on the GAO website at http://www.gao.gov.

If you or your staff have any questions concerning this report, please contact me at (202) 512-4841. Contact points for our offices of Congressional Relations and Public Affairs may be found on the last page of this report. Staff members making key contributions to this report are listed in appendix II.

Marie A. Mak
Director, Contracting and National Security Acquisitions

List of Addressees

The Honorable Patrick Leahy
Chairman

The Honorable Richard Shelby
Vice Chairman
Committee on Appropriations
United States Senate

The Honorable Ron Wyden
Chairman

The Honorable Mike Crapo
Ranking Member, Committee on Finance
United States Senate

The Honorable Patty Murray
Chair

The Honorable Richard Burr
Ranking Member
Committee on Health, Education, Labor, and Pensions
United States Senate

The Honorable Gary C. Peters
Chairman

The Honorable Rob Portman
Ranking Member
Committee on Homeland Security and Governmental Affairs
United States Senate

The Honorable Rosa L. DeLauro
Chair

The Honorable Kay Granger
Ranking Member
Committee on Appropriations
House of Representatives

The Honorable Frank Pallone, Jr.
Chairman

The Honorable Cathy McMorris Rodgers
Republican Leader
Committee on Energy and Commerce
House of Representatives

The Honorable Bennie G. Thompson
Chairman

The Honorable John Katko
Ranking Member
Committee on Homeland Security
House of Representatives

The Honorable Raúl M. Grijalva
Chairman
Committee on Natural Resources
House of Representatives

The Honorable Carolyn B. Maloney
Chairwoman

The Honorable James Comer
Ranking Member
Committee on Oversight and Reform
House of Representatives

The Honorable Richard E. Neal
Chairman
The Honorable Kevin Brady
Republican Leader
Committee on Ways and Means
House of Representatives

The Honorable Ruben Gallego
House of Representatives

Appendix I: Objectives, Scope, and Methodology

To identify the key characteristics of the Indian Health Service's (IHS) contract obligations made in response to the Coronavirus Disease 2019 (COVID-19) pandemic, we analyzed data available in the Federal Procurement Data System (FPDS) as of June 30, 2021.[1] We analyzed the FPDS data to identify the IHS area offices with the most contract obligations, as well as information such as the types of goods procured by these offices, rates of competition on awarded contracts, and characteristics of the vendors that were awarded contracts.[2] We assessed the reliability of FPDS data by

---

[1] For the purposes of this report, "contract obligations" means obligations on contracts that are subject to the Federal Acquisition Regulation, and does not include, for example, grants, cooperative agreements, loans, other transactions for research, real property leases, or requisitions from federal stock.

[2] For purposes of this report, competition rate is the percentage of total obligations associated with contracts awarded competitively. We calculated competition rates as the percentage of obligations on competitive contracts and orders over all obligations on contracts and orders annually. Competitive contracts included contracts and orders coded in FPDS as "full and open competition," "full and open after exclusion of sources," and "competed under simplified acquisition procedures," as well as orders coded as "subject to fair opportunity" and as "fair opportunity given," and "competitive set aside." Noncompetitive contracts included contracts and orders coded in FPDS as "not competed," "not available for competition," and "not competed under simplified acquisition procedures," as well as orders coded as an exception to "subject to fair opportunity," including "urgency," "only one source," "minimum guarantee," "follow-on action following competitive initial action," "other statutory authority," and "sole source." Even for contracts identified as noncompetitive, agencies may have solicited more than one source.

reviewing existing information about the FPDS system and the data it collects—specifically, the data dictionary and data validation rules. We determined the FPDS data were sufficiently reliable for the purposes of describing IHS's reported contract obligations in response to COVID-19. We primarily identified these contract actions and associated obligations related to the COVID-19 response by using the National Interest Action code.[3] We supplemented the use of the National Interest Action code by searching for "coronavirus" and "COVID-19" in the contract description field to identify a limited number of additional contract actions and associated obligations.[4] For the purposes of this report, we are focusing on IHS obligations for COVID-19- related medical products. In order to determine the increased obligations related to procuring COVID-19-related medical products, as presented in figure 3, we removed obligations for the pharmacy prime vendor (PPV) program from our calculations.[5]

To examine the contracting approaches IHS used to buy medical supplies and the challenges it faced in the award and administration of those contracts, we selected and reviewed the contract files for the five largest completed IHS contracts for COVID-19-related medical supplies as of January 25, 2021, when we began this review, based on FPDS data. The selected contract files account for 28 percent of obligations for the top product category—medical and surgical instruments, equipment, and supplies—as of June 30, 2021. During our review, we excluded one of these contracts because it was potentially the subject of an ongoing Office of Inspector General investigation. While the information we obtained from the selected contract files is not generalizable to all IHS contracts, the files provided examples of IHS

---

[3] National Interest Action codes were established in 2005 after Hurricane Katrina with the purpose of tracking federal procurements for specific disasters, emergencies, or contingency events. Based on a memorandum of agreement, the Department of Defense (DOD), the Department of Homeland Security (DHS), and the General Services Administration (GSA) are jointly responsible for when a National Interest Action code should be established and closed. DOD requests new or extended National Interest Action codes on behalf of the military departments and defense agencies, DHS requests new or extended codes on behalf of the civilian agencies, and GSA acts as the servicing agency by modifying FPDS.

[4] Our prior work identified some inconsistencies in the information agencies report in the contract description field. See GAO, *DATA Act: Quality of Data Submissions Has Improved but Further Action Is Needed to Disclose Known Data Limitations*, GAO-20-75 (Washington, D.C.: Nov. 8, 2019).

[5] IHS officials said that prior to August 2019, FPDS data included all obligations for the PPV program. IHS officials added that since August 2019, IHS has not reported PPV obligations for tribally-operated facilities in FPDS to ensure accurate reporting of IHS- specific obligations in FPDS.

procurements of COVID-19- related medical products. We also interviewed the cognizant contracting officers for these contracts to obtain their perspective on the contract actions and the circumstances surrounding the contracts. Additionally, we conducted interviews with officials at IHS headquarters, IHS's National Supply Service Center, located in the Oklahoma City area—which manages a large portion of IHS's COVID-19 contracts—to determine what challenges the COVID-19 environment presented and what contracting flexibilities IHS utilized to award contracts in response to the COVID-19 pandemic. We also asked officials about their contracting procedures during the interviews we conducted, and reviewed IHS's procurement policies in Part 5, Chapter 5, of the Indian Health Manual as well as portions of the Federal Acquisition Regulation.

We conducted this performance audit from January 2021 to October 2021 in accordance with generally accepted government auditing standards.

Those standards require that we plan and perform the audit to obtain sufficient, appropriate evidence to provide a reasonable basis for our findings and conclusions based on our audit objectives. We believe that the evidence obtained provides a reasonable basis for our findings and conclusions based on our audit objectives.

Appendix II: Staff Acknowledgments

In addition to the contact named above, Teague Lyons (Assistant Director), John Warren (Analyst in Charge), Jewel Conrad, Matthew T. Crosby, Suellen Foth, Stephanie Gustafson, Jeff Hartnett, Gina Hoover, and Robin Wilson made contributions to this report.

Index

A

access, viii, 16, 25, 29, 30, 148, 150, 152, 158, 167
accessibility, 158
accountability, 81, 111
accounting, 11, 17, 29, 44, 115, 164, 167
accounting standards, 167
acquisitions, 7, 12, 32, 34, 35, 36, 60, 176, 181, 186, 187, 188, 191
actuality, 75
adjustment, 156, 158, 162
administrative support, 105, 113
adverse weather, 117
aerospace, 119
agriculture, 10
Air Force, 101, 102, 118, 119, 120, 121, 133, 137
airports, 91, 100
Alaska, viii, 175, 176, 178
Alaska Natives, viii, 176, 178
American Indians, viii, 176, 178
American Red Cross, 118, 137
appropriations, 76, 150, 159, 160, 161
Appropriations Act, 83, 150, 152
assessment, 7, 10, 43, 46, 48, 50, 77, 97, 113, 159
assets, 9, 100
audit(s), 5, 8, 24, 29, 30, 57, 63, 77, 80, 85, 136, 150, 152, 174, 179, 196
awareness, 7, 30, 61, 191

B

banks, 10
base, 102, 105, 106, 108, 111, 113, 115, 120, 137, 159, 160, 168
benefits, 12, 101, 106, 127, 166, 167, 179
bilateral, 162, 163
blood, 83
business ethics, 11, 12, 20, 27
business model, 101
businesses, 76, 150, 153, 167

C

candidates, 94
CARES Act, vii, viii, 2, 5, 57, 73, 76, 77, 79, 80, 83, 84, 86, 96, 98, 99, 103, 110, 120, 121, 134, 136, 147, 148, 150, 152, 153, 159, 162, 190
cash flow, 102, 120, 133, 137, 153
certificate, 76
challenges, vii, 2, 3, 4, 5, 8, 28, 30, 33, 34, 37, 38, 39, 40, 43, 45, 46, 50, 52, 54, 57, 63, 75, 102, 109, 119, 164, 165, 167, 176, 178, 186, 190, 195
citizens, 45
cleaning, 101, 126, 133, 159, 160, 161, 168
clinical trials, 88, 94, 98
collaboration, 45, 51, 169
commercial, 21, 35, 82, 101, 117, 119, 187
commodity, 10, 32, 42
communication, 15, 25, 37, 38, 39, 45, 47, 50, 52, 100, 131, 133, 134, 162, 192
community, 10, 15, 35, 46, 159, 170

competition, 12, 14, 100, 181, 185, 186, 188, 194
competitive process, 94
compilation, 37
compliance, 128, 191
complications, 179
Congress, vii, viii, 28, 43, 73, 75, 76, 81, 82, 109, 127, 147, 150, 159, 160, 165
Consolidated Appropriations Act, 42, 150
construction, 9, 10, 11, 115, 117, 121
contamination, 40
contingency, 6, 15, 36, 44, 58, 92, 125, 135, 195
contract obligations, viii, 3, 5, 6, 16, 17, 18, 19, 20, 21, 30, 33, 47, 57, 58, 59, 79, 80, 86, 115, 116, 135, 136, 148, 151, 157, 160, 172, 174, 176, 177, 178, 182, 183, 184, 190, 194
contracting challenges, vii, 2, 4, 39, 43
cooperation, 119
cooperative agreements, 5, 6, 58, 178, 194
coordination, 4, 9, 15, 48, 50, 51, 52, 54, 122, 123, 126, 137, 149, 164, 165, 169
coronavirus, 5, 57, 58, 77, 116, 120, 130, 135, 150, 169, 181, 190, 195
cost, 14, 81, 82, 83, 84, 85, 99, 102, 103, 106, 111, 112, 121, 131, 153, 157, 160, 161, 162, 163, 167, 190
cost accounting, 81, 82, 163, 167
COVID-19 contract obligations, vii, 2, 6, 18, 20, 58, 59, 186
critical infrastructure, 158, 159
customers, 119, 164, 190
Customs and Border Protection, 132

D

data analysis, 79, 135
data collection, 15, 44, 46, 128
database, viii, 15, 43, 73, 74, 75, 91, 127
deaths, 76
decision makers, 51, 109, 110, 122, 123, 124, 127, 131, 134
Department of Energy, 147, 151, 156, 172
Department of Health and Human Services, 1, 24, 49, 61, 75, 76, 89, 95, 96, 101, 114, 116, 120, 121, 124, 130, 133, 137, 140, 175, 179, 192
Department of Homeland Security (DHS), vii, 1, 2, 3, 4, 6, 7, 8, 9, 14, 16, 20, 24, 26, 27, 31, 35, 37, 38, 39, 41, 42, 43, 46, 48, 50, 53, 54, 59, 60, 63, 74, 75, 78, 79, 82, 83, 84, 85, 86, 87, 88, 89, 90, 91, 93, 99, 101, 103, 109, 110, 114, 115, 116, 117, 122, 125, 126, 127, 128, 130, 131, 132, 133, 134, 135, 136, 147, 151, 154, 155, 157, 158, 159, 161, 163, 169, 172, 175, 195
Department of Defense (DOD), vii, viii, 1, 2, 3, 6, 7, 8, 9, 10, 14, 16, 20, 21, 24, 25, 31, 37, 38, 39, 41, 43, 46, 48, 49, 50, 53, 54, 58, 59, 60, 61, 63, 73, 74, 75, 76, 77, 78, 79, 81, 82, 83, 84, 85, 86, 87, 88, 89, 90, 91, 93, 94, 95, 96, 97, 98, 99, 100, 101, 102, 103, 104, 105, 106,107, 108, 109, 110, 113, 114, 115, 116, 117, 119, 120, 121, 122, 125, 126, 128, 130, 131, 132, 133, 134, 135, 136, 137, 147, 148, 151, 153, 154, 155, 156, 157, 160, 161, 162, 164, 167, 169, 172, 175, 195
detection, 101, 102, 132
deviation, 162
direct cost, 153, 164
disaster, 5, 9, 12, 13, 27, 28, 33, 36, 40, 43, 46, 51, 117, 186, 187
disaster relief, 117
disbursement, 77
disclosure, 167
diseases, 83, 100, 179
distribution, 33, 34, 38, 42, 44, 48, 52, 137, 190, 191
donors, 118
draft, 32, 54, 125, 169, 192
drugs, 17, 115

E

educational opportunities, 46
e-government, 92

emergency, vii, viii, 2, 4, 7, 9, 12, 13, 14, 20, 22, 28, 30, 31, 32, 33, 34, 35, 36, 44, 46, 47, 50, 51, 52, 53, 55, 60, 76, 84, 92, 110, 111, 147, 150, 176, 178, 183, 186, 187, 190, 191, 192
Emergency Assistance, 9, 12, 181, 186, 187
emergency planning, 35
emergency relief, 13
emergency response, 4, 32, 33, 36, 44, 47, 51, 52, 53, 55, 178
employees, viii, 43, 78, 111, 148, 149, 150, 152, 158, 159, 160, 162, 163, 166, 168
engineering, 9, 153
environment, 5, 47, 196
equipment, 10, 11, 22, 27, 35, 40, 61, 100, 115, 117, 118, 119, 159, 160, 168, 176, 177, 183, 187, 188, 190, 195
evidence, 8, 12, 27, 63, 80, 136, 152, 165, 174, 179, 196
exclusion, 194
execution, 108
executive branch, 128
exercise, 31, 42, 77
expenditures, 157
expertise, 38, 47, 48, 97

F

facility closures, viii, 148, 150, 152, 158
families, 76, 150
federal agency, 9
federal assistance, 9
federal contracting, vii, viii, 2, 3, 4, 5, 6, 7, 13, 15, 16, 17, 18, 22, 30, 37, 57, 59, 60, 61, 62, 73, 76, 77, 122, 148, 150, 176
Federal Emergency Management Agency (FEMA), 1, 4, 7, 9, 10, 14, 25, 26, 27, 28, 30, 34, 37, 38, 40, 43, 46, 47, 48, 50, 52, 53, 54, 55, 60, 62, 117, 178
federal government, 7, 9, 20, 28, 31, 33, 36, 58, 61, 79, 81, 91, 94, 102, 135, 151, 153, 167, 169, 172, 178, 185
federal law, 9
Federal Register, 179
financial, 11, 12, 24, 25, 29, 30, 53, 102, 120, 133, 137, 151, 153, 161, 163, 167, 168, 173
financial distress, 102, 120, 133, 137
financial relief, 153, 163
financial resources, 11, 29, 167
fiscal year, viii, 87, 104, 109, 115, 125, 148, 151, 153, 160, 172, 174, 185, 190
flexibility, 11, 19, 35, 44, 74, 81, 98, 99, 103, 189
food, 10, 33, 38, 44, 48, 52, 62
Food and Drug Administration, 40, 94, 188
fringe benefits, 153
funding, 33, 40, 93, 97, 99, 101, 102, 107, 108, 113, 117, 148, 149, 150, 152, 154, 155, 157, 159, 160, 161, 180, 190
funds, 20, 62, 77, 83, 102, 110, 154, 160, 179, 190

G

General Services Administration (GSA), 12, 75, 78, 92, 93, 109, 122, 123, 128, 131, 145, 151, 172, 175, 195
global economy, 76, 150
goods and services, vii, 2, 4, 6, 9, 10, 11, 13, 22, 27, 37, 39, 40, 45, 47, 52, 58, 73, 76, 122, 178, 186
government procurement, 107
governments, 31, 43, 46, 116, 119
grants, 5, 58, 84, 91, 120, 178, 194
growth, 118
guidance, vii, viii, 2, 5, 7, 14, 15, 22, 25, 26, 28, 30, 31, 33, 34, 35, 36, 38, 41, 52, 53, 60, 75, 79, 80, 92, 93, 114, 123, 124, 127, 128, 134, 136, 148, 150, 151, 152, 154, 156, 157, 159, 161, 162, 163, 164, 167, 169, 172, 192
guidelines, 159, 168
guiding principles, 169

H

health, 9, 10, 31, 42, 76, 83, 106, 125, 150, 153, 166, 168, 178, 179
Health and Human Services (HHS), vii, viii, 1, 2, 3, 4, 6, 7, 8, 9, 10, 11, 16, 20, 21, 24, 28, 29, 30, 31, 37, 38, 39, 40, 41, 42, 43, 44, 45, 46, 48, 49, 50, 53, 54, 55, 59, 60, 61, 63, 73, 74, 75, 76, 78, 79, 82, 83, 84, 85, 86, 87, 88, 89, 91, 92, 93, 94, 95, 96, 97, 98, 99, 101, 102, 103, 104, 109, 110, 113, 114, 115, 116, 117, 120, 121, 122, 123, 124, 125, 126, 128, 130, 131, 132, 133, 134, 135, 136, 137, 140, 175, 179, 181, 186, 187, 190, 192
health care, 9, 76, 150, 153, 178, 179, 180
health care system, 178
health condition, 179
health services, 178
homeland security, 110
Homeland Security (DHS), vii, viii, 1, 2, 3, 4, 6, 7, 8, 9, 14, 16, 20, 24, 26, 27, 31, 35, 37, 38, 39, 41, 42, 43, 46, 48, 49, 50, 53, 54, 55, 56, 57, 59, 60, 62, 63, 69, 73, 74, 75, 78, 79, 81, 82, 83, 84, 85, 86, 87, 88, 89, 90, 91, 93, 99, 101, 103, 109, 110, 114, 115, 116, 117, 122, 123, 124, 125, 126, 127, 128, 129, 130, 131, 132, 133, 134, 135, 136, 142, 147, 148, 151, 154, 155, 156, 157, 158, 159, 161, 163, 169, 170, 171, 172, 175, 193, 195
Homeland Security Act, 159
House of Representatives, 56, 57, 129, 171, 193, 194
Hurricane Katrina, 6, 40, 58, 135, 195
hurricanes, 4, 28, 36, 46, 162

I

Indian Health Service (HIS), v, viii, 31, 175, 176, 178, 180, 182, 183, 184, 185, 187, 188, 189, 190, 194
Indians, viii, 176, 178
individuals, 33, 42, 76, 118, 150, 165, 179
information sharing, 50
information technology, 153, 159
infrastructure, 120, 159
inspections, 40
institutions, 9, 104
integrity, 6, 11, 12, 16, 20, 24, 25, 27, 31, 59
intellectual property, 81, 98, 99
intellectual property rights, 81, 98
interagency coordination, 4, 46, 47, 48, 50
interface, 90
internal controls, 110, 131, 134
internal processes, 35
isolation, 22
issues, 9, 15, 25, 30, 33, 37, 42, 50, 102, 118, 167

J

justification, 94, 121, 186

L

labeling, 162
laws, 11, 74, 150
laws and regulations, 11
layoffs, 166
leadership, 43, 45
learning, 15, 51, 165
legislation, 80
life expectancy, 178, 179
liquidity, 168
loans, 6, 58, 153, 178, 194
low risk, 188

M

magnitude, 160
major disaster declaration, 15, 36
majority, 16, 18, 21, 31, 79, 80, 89, 93, 107, 109, 115, 135, 136
management, 13, 28, 31, 33, 34, 35, 36, 38, 74, 75, 79, 91, 96, 98, 103, 104, 105, 107, 110, 111, 113, 114, 117, 122, 123, 124, 126, 128, 131, 134, 170, 181, 187
manufacturing, 10, 40, 61, 74, 86, 88, 94, 95, 96, 97, 98, 125, 132, 133
marketing, 118

materials, 32, 37, 40, 81, 102, 153
medical, 9, 10, 22, 27, 31, 38, 40, 42, 45, 47, 48, 62, 83, 88, 106, 107, 111, 112, 113, 115, 120, 176, 177, 178, 180, 181, 183, 186, 189, 190, 195
memorandums of understanding, 10, 45, 48
methodology, 8, 80, 152, 179, 185
military, 81, 101, 106, 116, 119, 120, 121, 137, 159, 195
mission, 9, 10, 14, 31, 41, 44, 45, 48, 81, 83, 92, 106, 121, 158, 190
modernization, 160
modifications, 58, 59, 85, 100, 154, 156, 157, 162, 163, 184
morale, 166

N

narratives, 13
National Aeronautics and Space Administration, 147, 151, 156, 172
National Basketball Association, 102
National Defense Authorization Act, 82, 84
national emergency, 4, 9, 122, 148, 150, 153, 169, 181, 182, 185, 191
National Institutes of Health, 78, 83, 84, 87, 89, 91, 130
National Response Framework, 9, 15, 34
national security, 82
National Security Council, 50
natural disasters, 15, 125, 162
natural resources, 10
negative experiences, 15, 47, 51
negative outcomes, viii, 176
negotiating, 97, 113
negotiation, 106, 161
nonprofit organizations, 104

O

obstacles, 22, 34, 35, 36, 52, 53, 55
Office of Management and Budget (OMB), vii, 2, 15, 54, 55, 58, 60, 92, 111, 134, 147, 148, 149, 151, 152, 154, 156, 157, 164, 165, 169, 170, 172
Operation Enduring Freedom, 92
operations, 9, 13, 15, 20, 28, 36, 61, 125, 157, 159
opportunities, 128, 154, 181
organizational culture, 15
outreach, 53
oversight, viii, 35, 73, 74, 75, 77, 79, 81, 93, 97, 103, 113, 114, 122, 124, 125, 130, 134, 176
overtime, 37
ownership, 12, 151, 173, 174
ownership structure, 151, 173, 174

P

paid leave, v, viii, 5, 77, 147, 148, 149, 150, 151, 152, 153, 154, 155, 156, 157, 158, 159, 160, 161, 162, 163, 164, 165, 166, 167, 168, 169, 172, 173
paid leave reimbursement, v, viii, 5, 77, 147, 148, 149, 150, 151, 154, 159, 161, 162, 163, 165, 166, 168, 169, 172, 173
pandemic response, vii, 10, 33, 42, 43, 52, 73, 93
participants, 43, 82, 114
payroll, 153, 163
pharmaceutical, 75, 94, 98, 106, 175, 182
planned action, 126
policy, 7, 43, 50, 61, 79, 80, 91, 93, 111, 113, 117, 128, 134, 136, 149, 151, 153, 158, 165, 172, 181
policymakers, 91, 93
population, 27, 178
portfolio, 93, 98, 100
preparedness, 9, 10, 31, 43, 50
prescription drugs, 176
President, 15, 76, 111, 127, 150, 181
private sector, 9, 23, 47
procurement, vii, viii, 2, 13, 15, 31, 32, 36, 43, 46, 73, 74, 75, 76, 77, 79, 80, 81, 82, 83, 86, 87, 88, 90, 91, 92, 94, 97, 98, 99, 100, 102, 103, 115, 116, 122, 130, 134, 135, 136, 169, 177, 179, 186, 187, 188, 189, 196
profit, 10, 153

project, 82, 83, 97, 98, 106, 107, 113, 191
protection, 188
prototype, 81, 82, 83, 84, 95, 97, 98, 99, 100, 104, 105, 107, 126, 127, 131
public health, 4, 9, 10, 31, 42, 83, 84, 110
public interest, 75, 110
Puerto Rico, 46

Q

quality assurance, 113
questionnaire, 27

R

ratification, 31
raw materials, 37
reagents, 182
real property, 6, 58, 178, 194
recognized tribe, 179
recommendations, iv, 2, 15, 28, 41, 42, 43, 44, 51, 53, 54, 74, 122, 125, 126, 128
recovery, 10, 31, 51, 169
recruiting, 118
recurrence, 165
Reform, 57, 129, 171, 194
regulations, 7, 14, 15, 33, 60, 76, 80, 82, 85, 162, 163
reimburse, viii, 108, 148, 149, 150, 152, 154, 156, 157, 158, 159, 160, 164, 166
reliability, 6, 58, 59, 78, 79, 87, 88, 89, 91, 95, 104, 130, 131, 135, 151, 172, 178, 194
relief, 150, 154
repatriate, 45
research funding, 102
resilience, 43, 159
resolution, 43
resources, 7, 9, 11, 14, 22, 23, 24, 25, 26, 27, 28, 29, 30, 31, 34, 35, 36, 42, 43, 52, 53, 55, 60, 61, 125
respirator, 61
restrictions, viii, 148, 150, 152, 158, 187, 188, 189
revenue, 163
risk assessment, 7, 61
risks, 5, 25, 31, 33, 35, 75, 81, 85, 91, 110, 113, 114, 115, 121, 131
rules, 6, 58, 130, 135, 151, 172, 195

S

SACE, 9
safety, 94, 159, 166
savings, 100
scarcity, 47
Secretary of Agriculture, 53
Secretary of Defense, 54, 82, 84, 93, 98, 99, 109, 114, 122, 123, 124, 128
Secretary of Homeland Security, 9, 54, 122, 123, 124, 128
security, 31, 119, 150, 153, 158, 159, 167
security threats, 31
semi-structured interviews, viii, 7, 60, 148, 173
Senate, 56, 129, 170, 171, 193
services, vii, viii, 2, 4, 6, 9, 10, 11, 12, 13, 18, 22, 24, 27, 30, 34, 35, 37, 38, 39, 40, 45, 47, 48, 52, 58, 73, 76, 78, 79, 80, 85, 88, 105, 108, 111, 112, 113, 114, 116, 119, 122, 126, 130, 135, 153, 157, 159, 178, 179, 180, 181, 186, 188, 191
settlements, 161
small businesses, 13, 18, 153, 167, 181, 186
software, 153, 159, 176, 192
specifications, 85, 121
spending, 90, 91, 127, 153
stability, 150
staffing, 33, 40, 97
Stafford Act, 181
stakeholders, 42, 43, 46, 47, 52, 104, 128
statutory authority, 194
stock, 6, 58, 105, 108, 112, 178, 184, 194
storage, 38
structure, 106
subcontractors, viii, 148, 150, 152, 153, 167, 168
supplier(s), 10, 24, 168
supply chain, 30, 33, 37, 168

support services, 62, 103, 106, 107, 110, 111, 113
surveillance, 113
suspensions, 12

T

Task Force, 41, 44, 48, 50
taxpayers, 91, 110
technical comments, 54, 128, 169, 192
technical support, 48
territorial, 31, 43, 46
testing, 6, 10, 18, 58, 59, 78, 79, 100, 102, 106, 115, 130, 135
therapeutics, 10, 17, 83, 100, 103
time frame, 2, 3, 26, 28, 34, 36, 37, 39, 52, 53, 55, 58, 79, 80, 86, 93, 114, 135, 189
tracks, 91, 107
training, 30, 32, 36, 42, 46, 102, 113, 119, 167
transactions, 6, 58, 178, 194
transparency, 74, 75, 81, 92, 103, 110, 122, 126, 127, 128
transport, 62
Transportation Security Administration, 78, 81, 82, 83, 84, 99, 126, 130, 133
treatment, 25

U

U.S. Army Corps of Engineers, 2, 7, 9, 60, 61, 117, 120
U.S. Department of Agriculture, 2, 24, 62
United States, v, 1, 4, 56, 73, 129, 147, 170, 171, 175, 193
unsolicited proposals, 31
updating, 2, 36, 52, 53, 55, 114, 127
urban, 180, 190
urban areas, 180
USDA, vii, 2, 3, 6, 7, 8, 10, 16, 20, 24, 32, 33, 37, 38, 41, 42, 43, 44, 48, 53, 54, 59, 60, 63

V

vaccine, 10, 40, 61, 74, 78, 86, 88, 90, 94, 95, 96, 97, 98, 99, 103, 106, 132, 134
validation, 6, 58, 130, 135, 151, 172, 195
variations, 149, 164
vegetables, 10, 22
vehicles, 5, 40, 58, 94, 184
vendors, v, vii, 1, 2, 3, 4, 5, 6, 7, 11, 13, 16, 17, 18, 19, 20, 22, 23, 24, 25, 26, 27, 28, 29, 30, 31, 32, 33, 34, 35, 36, 37, 38, 39, 44, 48, 52, 53, 55, 57, 59, 60, 77, 176, 186, 189, 191, 194
vessels, 153

W

waiver, 120, 187
war, 106
Washington, 4, 5, 6, 7, 8, 33, 38, 40, 46, 51, 57, 58, 59, 61, 63, 77, 81, 85, 91, 92, 93, 95, 102, 110, 119, 150, 153, 164, 165, 167, 178, 179, 195
White House, 24, 38
work sites, viii, 148, 150, 152
workers, 153, 158, 159, 165, 178
workforce, 33, 35, 37, 48, 97, 148, 165, 166, 168
workload, 84, 192
World Health Organization (WHO), 150, 175, 181
worldwide, 119, 159